T0246947

Published 2024, USA.

First edition

eBook ISBN: 979-8-9873151-3-2

Print ISBN: 979-8-9873151-2-5

For further information, visit: WWW.WOLFEWELLNESS.CO

The FDA does not allow the natural health industry to make claims about their products without

scientific studies being performed that substantiate the claims. Although many facts herein are

scientifically referenced and/or evidence-based, this book is meant to educate you (the reader) about

natural remedies, herbs, supplements, and complementary therapies for wellness. Notwithstanding, this

should not be taken as a substitute for advice from a licensed health professional, who you should

consult in any matters requiring medical attention.

This information is intended for individuals 18 years and over. It is provided with the understanding that

the author is not engaged in the practice of medicine. None of the information or products discussed on

this site are intended to diagnose, treat, or cure any disease. Therefore, no guarantee, express or implied,

can be made. You are encouraged to verify for yourself and to your own satisfaction the accuracy of all

information, recommendations, conclusions, comments, opinions, or anything else contained within

these pages before making any decision based upon what you learn.

Table of Contents

Introduction

So you may have just come off the surgery table or recovery bed and you're not feeling at all like your old self ... and noticing that you may be a bit weaker than you were before.

I know what it's like.

After enduring my own surgical trauma in a very sensitive place many years ago, I found myself needing to get back on my feet and confidently get on with my life as soon as possible. My doctor was little help when he simply recommended rest, a handful of pain drugs, and antibiotics. So I needed to know how to recover quickly and to avoid side effects from modern drugs – which don't usually lead to regaining vibrant health. Since I already had some knowledge of natural and traditional remedies, I embraced this healing project and massively expanded my healing knowledge.

At the time, there were very few resources for this situation, so I had to scour diverse references, contacts, and resources. Since health has been my passion for the last 15 years, I was not starting from scratch. As I tapped into these new protocols, I recovered so quickly that during my first post-operation checkup, my doctor was amazed at my progress. He had to admit I was healing about twice as fast as most patients.

I realized I had something quite valuable to share with others seeking natural ways to speed their own recovery... hence this book I now share with you.

Our modern health landscape is dominated by Big Pharma, which pays millions of dollars to test their drugs in the hope of recouping their investment. No-one pays that

www.wolfewellness.co

money for testing natural remedies because it makes no business investment sense. Therefore, most natural remedies herein are based on the ancient scientific method of anecdotal (empirical) experiences. Said in another way:

> Empirical science, which is the scientific method of all original [traditional] cultures, is based on trial and error. That which has value is kept and employed. That which is found to have little or no value is dropped. In the empirical approach, that which is kept, is "tried and true".

Also, keep in mind that every person's body needs or reacts to any remedy in its own unique way. So, your underlying approach must be to test out these suggestions that are available, do-able, and applicable (empirically) - and then see for yourself which ones give you the results you seek.

How to best use this book

To get the most out of this book, scan each main healing category and consider the listed remedies that appeal to you (links for easy access are supplied wherever possible). While this book doesn't use pictures and eye-candy, it does provide concentrated, valuable content.

This book offers advice on many levels:
- Quick fixes
- Long term lifestyle changes
- Mild to acute pain relief
- Advice on helpful products
- Exercises and movements for recovery
- Professional resources and practice suggestions
- Further resources to continue on to super health!

The section called, *"Bringing it all together – recommended schedule"*, located at the end of this book, integrates most of the methods/remedies into a handy timetable. This gives

www.wolfewellness.co

you a quick understanding of what you should do and take at specific times in your recovery process.

Important notes on individual treatment effectiveness

- Each person may react a little differently to the same treatment (depending on the operation, injury, body types, genetics, environment, mental attitudes, lifestyle, etc); so when you try something, be aware of how your body responds. This also means that just because one person had miraculous results with a treatment doesn't necessarily mean that everyone will.

- Some treatments work synergistically; this means doing 2 or more things may make each treatment even stronger. This is a good reason to do as much as you comfortably can, and then consider adding more things as time goes on.

- There are 5 main healing areas to work with. The foundation of a holistic/alternative/natural approach is to improve all of them as much as possible. They are:
    - Diet – including supplements and herbs
    - Outer environments: weather, air, EMF/geopathic exposure
    - Inner environments: mental, emotional, spiritual, energetic
    - Physical activities, exercises, and therapies
    - Miscellaneous remedies

You can probably do at least one thing in each category. Remember the synergy of multiple remedies. Of course, these remedies should be fun because enjoyment is another important factor in healing... so don't stress over them. ☺

Energy levels

When recovering from surgery, you probably have less energy than usual. So how to increase your energy? Trying to "get" or "find" energy is like trying to grab a fistful of water. If you want water (energy) to sit in your hand, you have to first create the conditions under which it's possible -- in the case of water, keeping your fingers tightly together and your hand cupped while open will do the trick -- but trying to grab the water will not. It's the same thing with energy.

Energy isn't something you get or grab, but rather the by-product of certain conditions that allow it to accumulate in your body, and just show up in your life. If your health and attitude and body and mind are all aligned in the right way, there's nothing else for you to do but to feel energized. It's the natural "side-effect" of a healthy life -- it just comes with the territory. This is the wonderful by-product of holistic wellness for all aspects of your life: you increase the amount of positive energy, both physically and emotionally.

Your doctor

Although it may be too late for you to change doctors at this point, here is some brief advice. Most conventional doctors have little knowledge or regard for naturopathic and alternative health modalities because their training not only excludes that, but actively denigrates it. This means that when you start asking them specific questions about herbs, diet, or other natural remedies, you are likely to get little help. If you can find a doctor who supports natural remedies in addition to their conventional practice, then well done and consider yourself lucky.

General recovery notes (clinical)

Swelling (*hematoma)*

When you go home from the hospital you should have someone look at your wound progress (if applicable) on a daily basis. It is normal to have some fullness in your wound after surgery. This is a result of swelling or **hematoma**. A hematoma is an accumulation of blood that has occurred during and after your wound was closed. The surrounding area often becomes dark, bruised, stiff, and swollen. In most cases, your body will absorb this fluid with no additional concern.

If the hematoma is significant and has not begun to resolve after several days, your surgeon may consider removing the fluid by aspirating the wound. Other signs of concern will be redness or drainage from the wound. If the swelling is increasing, the wound becomes red / inflamed or you notice drainage, you should contact your surgeon or nurse for additional instructions.

During the first 2-7 days after surgery, your body uses inflammation to increase blood flow, clear debris, and limit infection. Therefore, a short/acute bout of inflammation is part of the healing process.

Healing cycle

Wounds heal in four basic stages:

1. **Wound sealing stage** – blood clots immediately following a breach in the skin to seal the wound and a subsequent scab forms. This starts within the first 5-10 minutes with a watertight seal normally

forming within 24 hours (large wounds may take longer).

2. **Inflammatory stage** – increased blood (both red and white cells) flows to and from the wound area making the wound area reddish, hot, and swollen... not to mention tender and painful! This stage starts after the wound is sealed (and not infected) and lasts for nearly a week. This is a challenging healing stage you will face and therefore much of this book is focused to help you past it. It is particularly important to not prolong this stage with the wrong diet, excessive use of NSAIDs (described later), and other aspects that you will soon understand. It may not seem like a big achievement, but simply <u>not</u> prolonging this stage is a big challenge for many patients who don't follow a healthy protocol for themselves.

3. **Tissue building stage** – new skin and new blood vessels form. This starts from the second day and takes an average of 4 weeks for moderate wounds with no complications. This is where you can make a positive difference in recovery time and coming back strong.

4. **Matrix building stage** – a matrix (mainly new collagen) forms for increased strength, stability, and overall integrity. This winding down stage can take from 24 days to 2 years.

Itching around the wound after a few days is a good sign that the healing process is underway.

www.wolfewellness.co

Diet

Whether you are recovering from organ surgery, oral surgery, bone surgery, laparoscopic surgery, tumor removal surgery, or any other - the right diet plan can have a big impact on the speed of your recovery and healing. Pain, bleeding, swelling, and surgery site inflammation will naturally occur at and around the surgery site. More specifically, by giving your body proper quantities of key nutrients, cleansing protocols, and avoiding the wrong foods can greatly assist in reducing the severity of the pain and swelling.

Water

Dehydration can lead to feelings of fatigue. If your body is imbalanced enough, it can lose its sense of thirst and even mistake it for hunger (for sweets, snacks, etc).

Substituting soda, coffee, black tea, or even fruit/veg juice for your water needs does not hydrate as well as water. Whereas certain herbal teas/extracts can contribute to your daily requirement, and even speed healing, black tea is acidic and diuretic.

Your water should be as pure as possible. That is to say, should not contain chlorine, farming pesticides, heavy metals, microbials, or other chemicals not properly filtered from the municipal recycling systems.

Quantity – since each body and physiological condition is unique, listen to your body's responses. Activity level, humidity, genetics, stress, and even gender (the Mayo notes that men need more water than women) are factors. Try drinking a single glass of water and check, for example, if it reduces false hunger pangs. Did you know that staying hydrated will help you to lose weight? If a person is

 www.wolfewellness.co

dehydrated, then their body may compensate by retaining excess water as a protective measure.

The U.S. National Academies of Sciences, Engineering, and Medicine determined that an adequate daily fluid intake is:

- About 15.5 cups (3.7 liters) of fluids a day for men
- About 11.5 cups (2.7 liters) of fluids a day for women

That may seem like a lot, but these recommendations cover fluids from water, other beverages and food. About 20% of daily fluid intake usually comes from food and the rest from drinks.

Other studies suggest about 6 - 8 glasses (8 oz) of just water per day. Also, except for the morning flush where you should have 1-2 glasses, water is better assimilated in smaller quantities more often; in other words, it's better to sip throughout the day rather than wait for hours then drink a lot in one go.

**How do you know you might need more water?
Here are 5 tell-tale signs:**

1. **Dryness:** dry lips, skin, eyes, and hair
2. **Inflammation:** skin rashes and burns, clogged pores leading to acne, red eyes
3. **Urine color:** your pee is dark yellow instead of light yellow (or clear)
4. **Constipation:** if you don't have a bowel movement for 1 full day or longer
5. **Sweat:** little to no sweat when exercising or in a hot environment
6. **Symptoms:** such as fatigue, dizziness, and confusion

www.wolfewellness.co

Timing – the best time to drink more water is first thing in the morning. This flushes the system after a long night. On the other hand, because water dilutes digestive juices, drink no more than a ½ cup within 15 minutes before a meal or no more than ½ cup within 60-90 minutes after a meal.

Electrolytes – Bio-science has confirmed that hydration is more effective when you take electrolytes with the water. That is to say, your body will absorb more water and benefit from it better when you make it more bio-available this way.

Here are some ways to increase the bio-availability of water:

- Take a pinch of salt with every glass you drink (approx 1/8 tsp per pint). Note that putting salt in your meal is not the same as having it with your drinking water. You can also just take a pinch and wash it down rather than mixing it in. If your stomach is a little uneasy with this at first, then drink the water more slowly. Moderate this if you're on a low-salt diet... these other additives can help.

- Add drops of a mineral concentrate such as:
    - Basic/alkaline: sodium chloride, potassium, calcium, and magnesium (**Note:** never drink alkaline water after eating as it neutralizes stomach acid and prevents digestion)
    - CELL FOOD, by NuScience
    - ConcenTrace, trace mineral drops (this gives additional benefits of

   mineralizing your body for improved
   healing)

  o There are other electrolyte drinks, but
   beware of those with added sugars or worse,
   artificial sweeteners

  o Add a few drops of peppermint essence or
   lemon juice

Temperature – modern tastes, especially American, prefer
ice-cold water. This puts a strain on your body because it's
much colder than your internal temperature and requires
your body to expend extra energy to warm it. This matter
is made worse if you drink the cold water just before a meal
because the cold water also paralyses your stomach, which
is not what you want just before putting food into it. After a
meal, your body uses heat along with gastric juices to help
digest the food; therefore, cooling it down with a glass of
ice-water demands extra energy and hinders digestion –
something you do not want. So at least room temperature
or even warmer. In Traditional Chinese and Ayurvedic
Medicines, warm/hot water is always preferred because it
imparts more energy to your body. Also keep in mind that
sipping warm/hot liquids is helps prevent cold/flu as it
maintains your internal body temperature.

Quality – don't trust your tap water unless you are sure it's
from a pure source. There are very few places in the world
where municipal water is wholesome. So if you don't
already have a water filter, get one now. Much is written on
how to best purify water, so to quickly sum it up:

Water distillers

  o They take out all minerals from tap water
   (you need all the minerals you can get) and

---

makes the water acidic. Tip: you want to eat and drink as much alkaline foods as possible. Read more about this in the *Alkalizing and blood (re) building* section. If you choose to drink this, then be sure to re-mineralize it or extended usage could be depleting.

Reverse osmosis

o They also take out most (of the few remaining) minerals and although not as bad as distillation, will make the water acidic. The reverse osmosis process wastes about 2x the amount of water that you can drink.

Bottled water

o Besides polluting the environment with plastic bottles and often having poor quality standards, poisonous dioxins from the plastic bottle often leach into this water. This is especially the case where a bottle of water is left in a hot place like inside a car, in the sunlight, or washing the bottle in hot-soapy water for reuse will also trigger this dioxin release.

Water softeners

o Water that has been *softened* (treated to replace the calcium and magnesium with sodium) is not fit to drink as it's too high in refined sodium.

Well or fresh spring water

o Lucky you if you can get this! Just be sure there is no run-off from any nearby farming chemicals.

Water filters

   o A good quality water filter is probably the easiest, cheapest, and best quality water you can get. There are many filters on the market, so here's one of the best that I have already tested, use, and recommend:

Drinking Water Filter
https://www.pureeffectfilters.com/filter-units/pure-effect-ultra.html#a_aid=RecoverFromSurgeryFast

Chlorine from the shower and bath

While we're on this topic, you should also consider getting a shower filter to remove all chlorine from your shower water. Why? The chlorine that your lungs absorb from taking a single shower will give you as much chlorine as if you had just drunk 8 glasses of water, which then adds to the toxic load on your body. Also, chlorine rapidly dries and ages your skin.

Shower Filter

https://www.pureeffectfilters.com/filter-units/pureshower-filter.html#a_aid=RecoverFromSurgeryFast

Salt

This is a very important – and widely misunderstood topic. It's also a big topic, so here's the summary version. People with high blood pressure are concerned about salt increasing this problem. Note that unrefined is much better at alkalizing and produces less blood pressure increase than common refined table salt. If you find that even these better quality salts trouble your blood pressure, than one can increase potassium, which will naturally lower the pressure.

Table salt – which is also what they use in most processed foods – has been ravaged in multiple refinery processes that remove useful trace minerals and then adulterated with toxic substances like bleach to whiten it, sugar to stabilize the added Iodine and as anti-caking chemical, moisture absorbents, Aluminum silicate as anti-caking chemical, heated under extreme heat levels in order to crack its molecular structure. However, if you can only find conventional salt, then at least choose *canning salt* as it has fewer additives.

Unrefined salt – is much better because this means the salt has come the way nature formed it. However, recent research is beginning to indicate that salt from freshly evaporated seawater may be more bio-compatible than that from ancient, deep underground deposits, which may have been influenced by intense heat. Along with supplying digestible and hard-to-get minerals, it greatly improves your stomach's own ability to produce hydrochloric acid and this is how it improves digestion. You can probably find some varieties of this in your local health food store; most important thing to look for is that it must say *unrefined*.

Alkalizing salt – a bicarbonate salt is the best salt to take in your drinking water because it combines the specific alkalizing sodium components such as (sodium bicarbonate, magnesium bicarbonate, potassium bicarbonate, and calcium bicarbonate). These salts are naturally occurring in all fluids of the body and as such help reduce acidity in the lymphatic, circulatory, and gastro-intestinal systems. Because they increase alkalinity, you may want to take them at least 10 minutes before or at least 60 minutes after an acidic meal (one that contains meat, diary, processed foods, or sugars; see the section on Alkaline Diet). This formula is called *pHour Salts* and available from Dr. Young: http://www.phmiracleliving.com/p-221-phour-salts-tm-454-grams.aspx?affiliateid=10152

Sweeteners

Refined sugars increase inflammation. The following list provides some wholesome alternatives. They are shown in order of increasing glycemic effect. Also understand that glycemic index is not the only index to measure the health affects. For instance, acusulfame, sucralose, aspartame, and saccharin are toxic (they are called *excitotoxins*):

- Stevia – ancient plant-based sweetener with no calories and no side effects

- Yacon syrup – Yacon syrup scores best in the Glycemic Index for sweeteners that are sugar-based because it derives its sweetness from fructooligosaccharides (FOS). Fructooligosaccharides are short-chain sugars that pass through the body's digestive tract as soluble fiber, without being absorbed or metabolized. A lower caloric count results from this process. FOS provides only about 1/3 of the calories as sugar (sucrose). The undigested portion of the FOS serves as a prebiotic providing nutrition for "good" bacteria found in the gut such as Bifidobacterium and Lactobacillus.

- Xylitol – a sugar alcohol that fights cavities; but over-doing it could cause a slight laxative effect

- Monk fruit sugar – the fruit's extract is used as a sweetener and is considered by the FDA as generally safe. The antioxidant, mogroside makes Monk fruit syrup sweet

- Honey (raw, unfiltered, organic) – more glycemic, but contains healing nutrients/enzymes that aid healing. Also useful for massaging onto the surface scar as explained in the *Massage* section of this eBook.

- Maple syrup – better is grade B (dark), which is less refined

Glycemic index expresses simply how quickly the carbohydrates contained in the ingested food turn into the digestive tract into glucose and it gets into the bloodstream. The expression of the Glycemic Index is relative because the GI index is 100 with glucose. However, this is not the highest value. There are sweeteners with a glycemic index greater than 100.

Here is a more complete list to compare of some common sweeteners:

Chart of glycemic indexes of sweeteners

Maltodextrin	110	Maltose	105	Dextrose	100
Dextrose	100	Glucose	100	Trehalose	70
HFCS-42	68	Sucrose	65	Caramel	60
Golden syrup	60	Inverted sugar	60	Refiners syrup	60
HFCS-55	58	Blackstrap molasses	55	Maple syrup	54
Honey	50	Sorghum Syrup	50	Lactose	45
Cane juice	43	Barley malt syrup	42	HSH	35
Coconut palm sugar	35	Maltitol	35	HFCS-90	31
Brown ruce syrup	25	Fructose	25	Galactose	25
Agave syrup	15	Xylitol	12	Glycerol	5
Sorbitol	4	Lactitol	3	Isomalt	2
Mannitol	2	Erythritol	1	Yacon syrup	1
Oligofructose	1	Inulin	1	Brazzein	0
Curculin	0	Glycyrrhizin	0	Luo Han Guo	0

www.wolfewellness.co

Miraculin	0	Monellin	0	Pentadin	0
Stevia	0	Thaumatin	0	Acesulfame K	0
Alitame	0	Aspartame	0	Cyclamate	0
Neotame	0	Sacharin	0	Sucralose	0

(www.fitnessmind.org)

Note: Agave syrup has become recently popular, however, my research has revealed that this is no better than High Fructose Corn Syrup...because this is just *High Fructose Agave Syrup*. Isolated fructose puts a great strain on the liver to process it into glucose...so let's not stress our liver any more than it already is.

It possible that when you crave sugar it is not really the need for sugar as much it is the need for salt. Eat some salt and your sugar cravings will go away with renewed and sustainable energy. Of course, the salt must at least be unrefined. Also, if the environment in your gut is over-run by bad bacteria and/or candida, then they are the ones craving sugar.

Fats & Oils

Some fats are healing and some are harming. It's crucial that you know the differences. Fats are categorized by what's called the Omega index. Also, raw fats help to repair tissue, while cooked fats are not as helpful. Our bodies have evolved off saturated/animal fats from the beginning, so beware of modern marketing that touts the benefits of highly refined fats.

Sources:

www.wolfewellness.co

Omega 3

Omega 3 is far too low in modern diets, so you will need to take special attention to increase this. As it turns out, plant-based omega 3 is not nearly as effective as the fish-based forms... Krill being the number 1 source. This should be taken twice daily. However, wait until about two to three days after surgery to ensure it does not interfere with normal blood clotting. (Fish oil has a very slight anticoagulant effect, which is mostly good—just not in the acute, post-trauma phase).

- Krill oil - most large ocean fish are high in mercury, and farmed fish have a toxic life. Therefore, a great source of fish-based omega-3 comes from Krill and you can find it here:

- Cod liver oil – includes the benefit of vitamins A & D. Be careful not to have too much vitamin A as it's fat soluble and doesn't eliminate quickly, like C. Also some cod liver oil could have mercury, so consider the source or use krill oil and then take separate vitamin D as needed.

- Salmon oil – If you prefer a less expensive option, this oil gives you great benefits at much less cost and is free of mercury

Here are some good food-based sources:
- Fish – small, oily fish like anchovies, mackerel, herring, catfish, and sardines along with wild salmon are best. Avoid big fish and

Mediterranean Sea fish due to high mercury levels. Also, high heat destroys omega 3, so consider lightly cooked or even raw sushi styles.

- Krill oil is the very best source of Omega 3:
- Avocados and their oil
- Borage oil – requires fish oil to balance GLA proportions
- Black currant oil
- Hemp seed oil
- Evening primrose oil – requires fish oil to balance GLA proportions
- Flaxseed oil – it's ok, but not nearly as good a source as fish oils
- Pumpkin seeds
- Walnuts and their oil
- Wheat germ oil
- Grass-fed beef – it's important to know that standard beef (grain-fed) has too much Omega 6 and you should avoid it especially during this healing time because Omega 6 worsens your inflammation.

Omega 6

Omega 6 is far too high in modern diets and it increases inflammation, so you should seek to minimize these oils and the foods that contain them. Here's a list of fats/oils that you should reduce/avoid as a lifestyle change:

- Processed oils – these are highly refined oils like shortening or margarine
- Hydrogenated oils

- Corn oil
- Soybean oil
- Cottonseed oil
- Canola (rapeseed)
- Safflower oil
- Sunflower oil
- Peanut oil

Cooking oils

The following oils are better for cooking because they do not break down as much under high heat (burn) as easily. This list is in order of best first.

1. Pure gee from organic grass-fed dairy
2. Butter from organic grass-fed dairy
3. Beef or pork fat (organic grass-fed)
4. Coconut (expeller pressed, organic, unrefined)
5. Palm
6. Avocado

List of Good Fats and Oils versus Bad

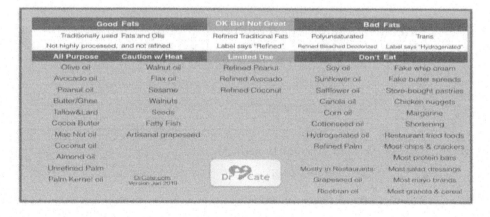

Good Fats		OK But Not Great	Bad Fats	
Traditionally used Fats and Oils Not highly processed, and not refined		Refined Traditional Fats Label says "Refined"	Polyunsaturated Refined Bleached Deodorized	Trans Label says "Hydrogenated"
All Purpose	Caution w/ Heat	Limited Use	Don't Eat	
Olive oil	Walnut oil	Refined Peanut	Soy oil	Fake whip cream
Avocado oil	Flax oil	Refined Avocado	Sunflower oil	Fake butter spreads
Peanut oil	Sesame	Refined Coconut	Safflower oil	Store-bought pastries
Butter/Ghee	Walnuts		Canola oil	Chicken nuggets
Tallow&Lard	Seeds		Corn oil	Margarine
Cocoa Butter	Fatty Fish		Cottonseed oil	Shortening
Mac Nut oil	Artisanal grapeseed		Hydrogenated oil	Restaurant fried foods
Coconut oil			Refined Palm	Most chips & crackers
Almond oil				Most protein bars
Unrefined Palm			Mostly in Restaurants:	Most salad dressings
Palm Kernel oil	DrCate.com Version Jan 2019	Dr Cate	Grapeseed oil	Most mayo brands
			Ricebran oil	Most granola & cereal

Protein

A variety of amino acids are required during wound healing and tissue regeneration, so ensure an adequate intake of protein. Although some protein may be obtained from non-animal sources, it's difficult to get the full spectrum of amino acids on a vegetarian diet... especially if your body needs to rebuild damaged tissues.

Pork is the most acidic and least beneficial meat, so you would do well eliminating that from your diet during the inflammatory stage. However, if you eat beef it is especially important during your recovery time that it's grass-fed. Otherwise, you'll be getting too much omega-6, which increases inflammation. The benefit of beef is that it has the most L-Carnitine, which is very beneficial for tissue and bone regrowth (see more details in the L-Carnitine section). Also, organ meat is much more nutritious than muscle meat... this is not a minor trivia!

A nice after-surgery recipe (note that since most non-organic chicken contains much omega-6, have this soup in moderation or alter it as needed with beef or fish if the inflammatory stage is noticeably slow/painful).

Healing organic chicken soup with veggies and grains:

- A small chicken, bought organic at the local farmers market, with gizzards and all.
- 1 lb carrots
- 1 package celery (about 10 stalks, probably a little over a pound)
- 1 large onion
- 1 head of broccoli

- 1 large sweet potato, including peel
- bay leaf
- 2-6 cloves of garlic – added after cooking
- salt (unrefined; see Salt section)
- pepper – cayenne & black
- 2 tsp. turmeric
- 4 oz fresh ginger
- other spices as desired – fresh is better
- 10 oz frozen package of peas
- 1 lb dry grain - see the grain section

1. Rinse the chicken. Place in large soup pot, fill three-quarters full with water and bring to a boil. Simmer covered for 1 & 1/2 hours (if frozen, then 2 hours). If the meat is not chicken, then not necessary to cook as long because only chicken imparts certain healing qualities after long boiling.

2. Spoon out excess fat from the top (only if you're sure you need to reduce fat content).

3. Add salt and black pepper to taste.

4. Add carrots, celery, peas, onion, broccoli, sweet potato, turmeric, and ginger. Stir in bay leaf and oregano, then cook for another 30 minutes.

5. Add fresh basil, fresh parsley, fresh garlic, and cayenne pepper to taste, then serve.

Food – general concepts

Raw foods

The amount of raw food in your diet is one area that has well-supported pros and cons, so this section will help you work out what's best for you.

www.wolfewellness.co

When you move your diet towards more organic raw vegetables, your body will simultaneously get more of these building blocks needed to rebuild and begin to slowly detox.

On the other hand, eating a diet of mostly cooked and, especially, pre-processed food lacks many essential nutrients and enzymes -- particularly on the pancreas since it has to produce massive quantities of digestive enzymes since they no longer come with the food itself. The less digestion that takes place before food reaches the small intestine, the greater the stress placed on the endocrine system. Is it any wonder that the incidence of diabetes is exploding in the developed world? If your diet consists of predominantly cooked and processed foods, then supplemental digestive enzymes are the "sine qua non" of minimal good health.

On the other hand, an advantage of cooking is that makes some foods easier to digest and may release certain nutrients. If you are accustomed to very little raw food, then you will need to make the transition to increase raw slowly and according to your body's response to it. In other words, if a big salad (or any new food for that matter) gives you gas, indigestion, heavy feeling for many hours afterwards, diarrhea/constipation, bad taste in the mouth, or other feelings of discomfort, then reduce it until your body adjusts. If your body does not adjust after a couple of weeks, then that food may not be the right thing for you at that time.

The amount of raw food in your diet is where different philosophies disagree. Also, different people do have different metabolisms, nutritional needs, and digestive ability. The general goal to strike a balance is to have 20 - 40% of your diet raw. Here's an example of a more detailed breakdown:

www.wolfewellness.co

- 30% - raw vegetables (includes sprouted beans/seeds)
- 10% - raw fruit
- 35% - cooked veg (see Note 6)
- 10% - cooked, soaked, sprouted, or (best is) fermented grains
- 15% - animal products (meat and raw dairy depending on individual needs)
- **Note 1** – when you are eating mostly cooked foods, it is so beneficial to take a digestive enzyme with the meal to "put-back" those enzymes that were lost in cooking. This also makes it easier on your body in general because it won't have to work so hard to generate the required enzymes.

- **Note 2** – again, listen to your body. If you don't feel well after eating something, then avoid it – for a while. If it's a wholesome and alkalizing food, then try again a few days later if you want to. Either it's not right for your body type or not right at this time (maybe it makes you detox too quickly).
- **Note 3** –when in recovery mode, you will need more proteins to rebuild and more raw foods to cleanse/detox.
- **Note 4** – produce should be organic whenever possible. If not, then wash them with a veggie-wash fluid to at least remove surface pesticides and waxes (this wash is available at most health-food stores)
- **Note 5** – when cooking food, steam-frying is the healthiest option rather than boiling or

just frying. Cooking with both water and oil brings out the full spectrum of nutrients. Never eat burnt meat.

- o **Note 6 –** in a cold climate or season, raw foods may be too cooling, so use less at this time.
- o **Note 7 –** a superior way to have raw food is to make veggie or fruit smoothies using a blender or food processor.

Food combining

Although many books have now been written on this, here is 80% of the benefit reduced to a few quick pointers:

- o Eat fruits on an empty stomach at least 15 minutes before other foods...especially melons. However, apples and pineapples contain digestive enzymes and so can be eaten after meals. They are the only exceptions to this rule...and in moderation.
- o Avoid eating meat and starchy foods (grains and starchy veggies like potatoes) at the same time. If you do eat meat in the same meal, then have the meat before any starchy food enters your mouth. This allows the stomach to use its full acid resources to start digesting the meat. Otherwise, the digestion starts on the starch in the mouth and uses more alkaline elements to digest the whole meal...which does not break down the meat as it requires hydrochloric acid (HCL) in the stomach.
- o Eat dairy sparingly and when you do, it should be raw and even better if not mixed with anything else. Butter and ghee don't have this issue.

o If have a meal with both meat and starchy carbs, there is a little-known fact that can still help very much. The stomach digests foods in layers – working on the first layer first. This means that if you eat all the meat by itself, the stomach can work on this with its HCL. Thereafter, you can combine and digest the rest of the meal (starches, fats, complex carbs like vegetables) without as much digestive conflict.

Alkalizing and blood (re) building

This can be a very beneficial diet to embrace, which will *help you attain all your health goals.* This diet is especially important if your surgery was the result of a disease (such as cancer or a troubled organ) as opposed to a mechanical issue (such as broken bone, accidental damage, or cosmetic surgery). True to the summary nature of this eBook, here is a basic understanding in a nutshell…

Your body will be healthier, heal faster, and last longer If It is more alkaline. It is designed to be alkaline because when it is running (when you are alive), it produces acids that need to be neutralized - think of hydrochloric acids used in digestion and lactic acids that make muscles sore after exercise. So you need to put as much alkaline food into your body as possible and minimize acidic foods and inner processes. An acidic body is a breeding ground for many diseases and cellular dysfunctions.

The most alkaline foods are fresh, raw (or lightly cooked), organic vegetables and sprouts. The most acidic foods are vinegar (pure acid), refined sugar, black tea, coffee, alcohol, soft drinks (sodas), and cooked/processed red meats.

Another aspect about alkalizing is emotions. Negative emotions produce acid in the body and positive ones produce alkaline. In other words, when you're happy and peaceful, your body will be more alkaline, and thus stronger and healthier. To better deal with this aspect, see the section on *Mind-body connection*.

Paleolithic diet

Our ancestors (all of them for the last 2 million years or thereabouts) ate a diet mostly consisting of wild fruits, nuts, seeds, vegetables, insects, and animals...all raw! Not surprisingly, raw food is far healthier than cooked foods. For more info on the Paleolithic diet, just search the web or get a book on it. Suffice it to say, you should strive to make your diet at least 2/3 raw. This includes raw animal products (eggs, dairy, and meat). It is important to understand a few things when eating raw animal products (and this is where a full book will give you the details to do it properly):

- o The media and "modern" advice has scared people into thinking that all raw animal products are dangerous. Well if that's the case, how did we survive for several million years on them?

- o Cooked and pasteurized foods can still carry the same pathogens as raw foods.

- o There are certain precautions to take that will almost eliminate the risk with raw foods. Here are a few to get you started:

- o Eggs: buy organic, free-range. Wash the outside shell with veggie-wash. When you break them open, smell the contents before pouring out (they should smell fresh; otherwise, don't eat). Chilled eggs will smell fresher than they should; so leave the eggs out in room temperature for an hour before eating to know their true smell. Obviously if they look strange inside (black spots and such), then don't eat.

- o Meat: poultry is in fact too risky to eat raw. Red meats should be organic, free-range, and grass-fed. Rinse the meat well. A further precaution would be to just sear the meat in a frying pan for about 1 minute per side (also sere the edges). This will kill any surface bacteria and leave most of the meat in a raw state. As long as it's not pre-ground, there is little chance of bacteria/pathogens beneath the surface.

- o In fact, when your digestive system is stronger, it can handle most bacteria without much problem. If you suspect that you're not ready for the Paleo diet, just avoid overcooking (burning) the meat.

Metabolic typing

With these previous principles in mind, there is another aspect to consider. Some people have a stronger protein (meat) requirement while others are better off with a carbohydrate (vegetarian) diet and the rest are in between (mixed). This is due to your metabolic type, ancestry, lifestyle, and even more factors. You can learn about your own optimal balance by researching your metabolic type. However, metabolic typing is not an exact science, so you should follow your body's intuition (not sugar cravings) to fine-tune this plan. To learn more about discovering what is best for your type, click below:

Metabolic Typing http://products.mercola.com/nutritional-typing/?aid=CD426

Chew your food

Some health gurus state it this way: chew your liquids and drink your solids. This means that you should chew your solid food so well that it becomes a liquid and you should even chew your liquids a bit to begin their digestion in the mouth and alkalize them. If this seems like too much trouble, then you must understand that digestion begins in the mouth. That's how we are designed. If you bypass that by rushing this step, then you seriously reduce you body's ability to absorb the nutrition that it so desperately needs. This is such an ancient topic, that if you need more convincing, a quick web search will reveal mounds of scientific reasons and evidence to support this.

So exactly how many times should you chew? Well that depends on the type of food and the efficiency of your own set of teeth. A good rule of thumb for the minimum chewing is as follows: if you <u>can</u> tell what kind of food you are eating from the texture of the food in your mouth (not the taste), then you haven't chewed it enough. For example, if you are chewing broccoli and you run your tongue over the stalk inside your mouth and can tell that it is still a stalk or over the floret and you can still tell that it is still a floret, then don't swallow. You need to keep on chewing until you can't tell the stalk from the floret. However, with respect to doing this better, you should also chew mushy things as well – like mashed/pureed veggies, soups, and such.

Many people substitute chewing for just washing their food down with a big beverage. This is not a good idea because it dilutes the stomach's digestion process and can make you feel bloated. A half-cup of water before and can help some people; otherwise, avoid drinking anything more within 10 minutes of a meal and not until 45-60 minutes afterwards. Since your digestion also requires heat in it's process, avoid having a very cold desert (ice cream) following a big meal.

Chewing well also goes hand-in-hand with creating a peaceful and grateful environment around a meal. Never eat when you are upset or your emotions are negative. To reduce negative emotions quickly, use the Sedona Method or Emotional Freedom Technique.

Flavors

The **Chinese** and **Ayurvedic** health systems understand that we need to notice and balance the types of flavors we are consuming. There are 6 basic flavors:

- Sweet
- Salty
- Sour
- Pungent (spicy)
- Astringent (contains tannins)
- Bitter

Modern diets are too excessive in salty and sweet flavors and too deficient in the bitter and astringent flavors, which are especially helpful for your recovery process. Their natures are antibiotic, antiseptic, anti-inflammatory, reduces bleeding, and also clears and cleanses the mind and emotions. Because it improves digestion, it will help you gain more rebuilding nutrition from everything else you eat.

Bitter foods helps relieve mucus, pus, and watery accumulations; such foods are also slimming. Western herbalism which has long touted various bitters (gentian, dandelion, aloe vera, goldenseal, etc.) for treating a wide range of conditions predominantly associated with the liver. Bitters are purifying and detoxifying and they help to remove poisons from the blood. Many bitters are germicidal, bactericidal, and anti-inflammatory. The best known herbal formula is Swedish Bitters. Of the **culinary** spices which are bitter, **turmeric** is perhaps the most widely used; **Coriander** leaves (aka **Cilantro**) is another.

Before you panic about having to eat bitter foods, know that there are many vegetables in the **bitter class**, which do not really taste bitter. Here are some examples:

- o dark leafy green vegetables like spinach, chard, kale, and dandelion
- o rhubarb
- o bitter melon
- o Herbs: see above paragraphs for medicinal and culinary herbs

Astringent foods containing tannins are chiefly useful in reducing irritability. They are slightly anesthetic and therefore calming, but they also reduce sensitivity. The astringent herbs perhaps best known in the West are sage and St. John's wort.
Here are some examples of **astringent foods**:

- o cruciferous vegetables: broccoli, cauliflower, kale, brussel sprouts
- o okra
- o beans & lentils
- o unripe bananas & persimmons
- o cranberries
- o pomegranates
- o Herbs: parsley, basil, saffron, turmeric

So increasing these vegetables should be helpful. Obviously you should also minimize the pasta, cheese, pastries, junk food snacks, and sweets. In the spirit of this book, however, I want to open your eyes to this important aspect and so

 www.wolfewellness.co

give you more understanding about your diet. To further benefit your immediate and specific needs from these 2 ancient and powerful systems, I recommend you find a local and trusted practitioner.

Specific foods

Garlic

Nature's most excellent general anti-microbial (like an anti-biotic without any of the bad side-effects). Even Western medicine acknowledges garlic's amazing ability to help lower cholesterol and reduce the risk of further heart attacks in cardiac patients. It's also known for its ability to stimulate the immune response along with its antibiotic properties. It is beneficial to the nervous system and is especially useful in lowering hypertension (proven in laboratory tests). Garlic improves blood circulation, is alkalizing, and is very useful as an expectorant for lung congestion and infections. It can also have a stimulating effect. This means if you're feeling generally sluggish it will be energizing, but if you're mostly agitated, it may not be the right thing for you. If you're not sure about it, just try it and see. Because this is a benign and natural food, you can't go far wrong with it.

The best way to benefit from this food is eating the raw cloves. The active ingredient is destroyed within one hour of smashing the garlic. In other words, don't cook them, don't store them as crushed leftovers, and don't waste your money with 98% of the extracts/capsules for sale because very few manufacturers know how to preserve the holistic properties. So here are some suggestions to eating this powerful food:

- o Start with a single clove with food because some people may feel a little stomach upset the first few times

- ○ Crushing it into your salads is a good way
- ○ If using in cooked food, then add this after the dish is done cooking – just before serving. This will preserve the medicinal qualities
- ○ Don't have this before a surgery or for the first few days following because it can have an anti-clotting effect on the blood. Furthermore, if already on blood thinning drugs like warfarin (coumadin), garlic is not a good idea since it would add to the drug's effect
- ○ There is only one formula that I've personally felt strong results from and it combines the other raw essences of cayenne, oregano and several other powerful anti-microbials

Sprouts

This is a very simple food but is probably one of your best sources of potent recovery nutrition. When a seed, bean, nut, or grain begins to sprout there is tremendous change in its character and nutritional value to you. Whereas unsprouted foods have built-in resistance to enzymes (which allows them to last on the shelf for so long), they virtually explode with enzymes and life force when they begin to sprout. If you don't already have a sprouter jar, then here is an easy and effective solution:

If you at least soak your seeds, beans, nuts, and grains for about 8 hours before eating/cooking, then it is better than nothing, as it removes phytic acid, but not as good as sprouting.

Bone Broth

Something just coming into the public attention and grocery shelves is bone broth. This is an excellent way of

www.wolfewellness.co

getting a wide array of nutrients and minerals that are bio-available. As with most things, organic is better here as well.

Super Healing Drink

To get enough of the right healing nutrients into your body, the following drink will make up for most dietary deficiencies... it is your magic elixir. Combine these ingredients into a shaker jar or blender (shaker jars may not mix quite as well, but they don't beat up the nutrients quite so hard as blenders and are therefore a bit healthier).

- 1 glass of pure water and/or bone broth
- 1-3 tsp green food concentrate
- 1 scoop of whey concentrate powder
- Glutamine
- 1-2 tsp aloe vera concentrate or gel
- Sweeten to taste with Stevia

Supplements

Vitamins

Before using vitamins after surgery, consult with your doctor to make sure they don't interfere with any medications you may be taking.

A

- This is known for boosting the immune system, which can help ward off infection after your surgery. Furthermore, vitamin A encourages new cell growth, which is essential for a rapid recovery. Just be careful not to overdose on this (or any other oil-based vitamin). It is also plentiful in butter. Most brands of cod liver oil have too much vitamin A.

B

- o Although B12 & B6 are helpful for increasing energy (and paradoxically improving sleep), it's usually better to take the entire complex as they synergistically improve each other. An exception would be if you really have chronic low energy, then a B-12 oral spray could solve this deficiency directly. Take during the day, not before bed.   B-12 oral spray http://products.mercola.com/vitamin-b12-spray/?aid=CD426

C

- o Increase your vitamin C intake up to 5000 mg per day 3 days before, then to 10,000 mg per day after surgery. Medical practitioners say that vitamin C boosts your body's immune function, reduce general inflammation, and help it heal. Buffered vitamin C as that is not so acidic and is absorbed better.

D

- o In just the last couple of years, science is starting to uncover the secrets of this vitamin. The next 3 or so bullets get a bit scientific, but it's good for you to understand that this vitamin is extremely important.
- o It's important to realize that vitamin D is not "just a vitamin," but rather the only known substrate for a potent, pleiotropic (meaning it produces multiple effects), repair and maintenance seco-steroid hormone that serves multiple gene-regulatory functions in your body.

As one Dr. Robert Heaney explains in his lectures, each cell in your body has its own DNA library that contains information needed to deal with virtually every kind of stimulus it may encounter, and the master key to enter this library is activated vitamin D.

- For example, memory ductile cells in the breast need vitamin D to access DNA that enables the response to estrogen.
- So naturally, without sufficient amounts of vitamin D, your cells cannot access their DNA libraries and their functions are thereby impaired.
- This is why vitamin D functions in so many different tissues, and affects such a large number of different diseases and health conditions. So far, scientists have found about 3,000 genes that are upregulated by vitamin D.
- Receptors that respond to the vitamin have been found in almost every type of human cell, from your brain to your bones. And researchers keep finding health benefits from vitamin D in virtually every area they look.
- Vitamin D Deficiency May Radically Hamper Your Overall Health. Just one example of an important gene that vitamin D up-regulates is your ability to fight infections, including the flu. It produces over 200 anti microbial peptides, the most important of which is cathelicidin, a naturally occurring broad-spectrum antibiotic.
- Optimizing your vitamin D levels can also help you to prevent as many as 16

different types of cancer including pancreatic, lung, breast, ovarian, prostate, and colon cancers.

- o But perhaps most important to note is that vitamin D can lower your risk of dying from any cause, according to a new European meta-analysis published in the Archives of Internal Medicine in 2007.
- o Sunshine is the best source (see the section on *Sun* for dosage).
- o However, if you live in an area where you can't get much sunshine directly on your bare skin, then you should either supplement orally or use a full spectrum sunbed.
- o Also, since most people are critically low in this important vitamin, the best protocol to restore and then maintain D levels is (yes, it seems like a very big dose, but this works best; if you're concerned about this, you can test your reaction to large doses by starting with only 10,000 iu for a few days):
  - ▪ Take 50,000 IU 1x/day for 3 consecutive days
  - ▪ After that, to maintain, take 50,000 IU 1x/week
  - ▪ Vitamin D is better absorbed if you take vitamin K along with it
- o Oral Vitamin D spray : http://products.mercola.com/vitamin-d-spray/?aid=CD426

- o Sunbed : http://products.mercola.com/tanning-bed/?aid=CD426

E

- o Add an extra dose of vitamin E as you recover from your surgery. Vitamin E is

   www.wolfewellness.co

known for promoting healthy skin and hair growth; so it can help heal your wound faster. It also enhances fish oil and Glutamine supplements. Be sure to use a brand with naturally derived mixed tocopherols. Vit E
http://products.mercola.com/vitamine/?aid=CD426

K

- o A key nutrient important for blood clotting, which is vital for wound sealing. Abundant in fermented foods (sauerkraut, sourdough, miso, kim-chi, etc) and leafy green vegetables; it is then synthesized by bacteria in your intestines. This is another reason to avoid antibiotics as much as possible as they kill off these good bacteria. See the probiotics section to replenish these.

Minerals

With modern farming and even worse – modern diets – it's difficult to get your required nutrients. When you need to heal, supplementing your diet with vitamins and minerals is even more necessary.

Colloidal trace minerals

Because of commercial farming, modern produce is nearly devoid of the minerals that they should have and that your body should have. Unless you have been eating top standard organic produce for the last 10 years, your body is probably deficient in multiple minerals. During this healing phase, it is especially important that your body gets these basic building blocks. The colloidal form of minerals just means that they are such tiny particles, that they are suspended in water. This allows your body to absorb a much higher percentage of what you give it. In other words, if your body can only absorb 5% of the 100 mg in your mineral tablet, then it's only getting 5 mg. However, if it can absorb 95% of a colloidal mineral containing 20 mg of these minerals, then it's getting 18 mg...and in a form that is easier for it to digest (this also means less energy taken away from you).

Colloidal silver

This is another one of nature's wide-spectrum antibiotics. There is also something called silvadine, which is used as a topical burn treatment. Colloidal silver is a powerful antibiotic for both internal and topical use. It can treat drug-resistant staph, tuberculosis and the bird flu. In Africa, it is used to treat just about everything, including AIDS, hepatitis, malaria, cholera, and pneumonia. It can be used topically to treat burns, wounds, thrush and other skin infections.

Use a 5-parts-per-million concentration, at a dose of one teaspoon three to four times per day. There have been rare instances of silver overdose called agryria, which is an irreversible blue/gray discoloration of the skin. However, this is from ingesting silver salts, not colloidal silver – and in excessive quantities (when using as an internal/systemic antibiotic, you usually only need a couple teaspoons per day for no more than a week or two). Carefully research the product you are buying for is strength and purity and follow the directions for usage to the letter. Also, bear in mind that this will also kill off good bacteria (just like any antibiotic) in your digestive tract, so after finishing a course of this remedy, you should re-populate your good gut bacteria with pro-biotic supplements and (fermented) foods.

Selenium

This lesser-known trace element helps the wound itself to heal. If you experience muscle spasms/cramps, it can mean that you are deficient in this. Your multiple vitamin should contain 100-200 mcg per day.

Zinc

Although it's considered only a trace element, zinc is very helpful in tissue healing and forming connective tissue. Also, it greatly improves your immune system. You should have this in your multiple vitamin in the range of 15-45 mg per day. Additionally, if you have a sore throat

www.wolfewellness.co

from cold or flu, zinc lozenges can quickly cure the throat and help with other cold/flu symptoms.

Zinc is much more effective when taken with Quercetin.

Multi vitamin & mineral formula

Since your body uses some vitamins or minerals to help absorb others, it's always better to get them all at the same time and in the widest combination. This is how they come in whole foods...hence, multiple vitamins make good sense. However, not all multiples are equal. Many use inorganic sources and therefore do not absorb well. In fact, these cheap multiples usually only deliver from 0.3 – 5% of what they contain. This is very important when you're trying to maintain the right levels of certain nutrients. Also, as mentioned elsewhere in this eBook, most tablets contain Magnesium Stereate, which not only hinders nutrient absorption, but also suppresses your immune system. Here is an excellent whole food derived multi that satisfies these difficult criteria. Note that it deliberately lacks vitamin D because individual needs will vary widely for this and it's best not to overdose on D. Wholefood Multivitamin
http://products.mercola.com/multivitamin-vital-minerals/?aid=CD426

Herbs

Here is general advice for obtaining higher quality herbs:

o   Select the best quality you can find because it will make a difference – especially when you want them for medicinal purposes. Quality starts with organic, wild-crafted, non-irradiated (most herbs are best when whole powder rather than extracts).

o   Some herbs/spices need to be cooked to release their healing qualities. However, the aromatic (salad) herbs like parsley, basil, dill, coriander are better raw or only lightly cooked so as to preserve their essential oils.

- If you do take extracts (whether capsule or tincture), the strength of most commercial brands is only on average a fraction of what they should be for the effect you need. Because of the great variance in different brands and your individual needs, the only way to know is to test on yourself by gradually increasing the dose until you either feel the right effect or otherwise reach your limit. Since herbs are holistic, it's probably difficult to overdose - as with pharmaceutical drugs.

If you choose to use the liquid/extract form, then be aware that they can have a very strong flavor. A good method for taking these extracts is the "shot glass technique." Pour only about 2 ounces of water/juice into a glass, then add all your liquid extracts. Have another glass of water/juice close by. Drink the herbal tonic right down then quickly chase it with the plain liquid.

Astragalus

Take this herb to increase your white blood cells. These are the guys who clean up the trash and repair your body; so you want lots of them. Note that if your body is generally warmer than others (hot-blooded), then this may not be right for you as it tends to slightly increase heat in the body – it's a warming herb, like ginger or ginseng.

Boswellia

Also known as boswellin or "Indian frankincense," this herb contains specific active anti-inflammatory ingredients, referred to as boswellic acids that animal studies have shown significantly reduce inflammation. This is one of my personal favorites as I have seen it work well with many of my rheumatoid arthritis patients

 www.wolfewellness.co

Cayenne

A common culinary spice, this herb helps to strengthen the effectiveness of all other herbs. It also improves circulation, is a general anti-microbial and enhances digestion. To use it for digestion, start off with a ½ tsp in 1-2 oz of water about 5 minutes before a meal. You can work up to several teaspoons as you see the good results. Of course, you may also develop a taste for this potent condiment. However, do not cook it or it will lose its beneficial properties and become a little toxic.

Cayenne (Cream)

Also called capsaicin cream, this form helps to alleviate pain by depleting the body's supply of substance P, a chemical component of nerve cells that transmits pain signals to the brain.

Meadowsweet

Also known as Filipendula almaria, is a herb which has been used for centuries by herbalists to treat fever and pain. Modern science reveals that this herb contains salicylates - a natural chemical similar to the pharmaceutical aspirin. Unlike, aspirin, however, Meadowsweet has pain relieving and anti-inflammatory properties without side effects such as stomach ulcers and the risk of Reynaud's Disease, associated with the use of pharmaceutical aspirin.

Ginger

This Anti-Inflammatory herb is anti-inflammatory and offers pain relief and stomach-settling properties. Fresh ginger works well steeped in boiling water as a tea or grated into vegetable juice. Powder capsules are also available, but I recommend using the fresh root.

Oregano

Check your spice shelf. Wild oregano and oregano oil both fight bacterial, viral and fungal infections, along with boosting your immune system. Use oregano to help fight systemic and skin infections. The oil essence is even stronger; apply it topically or dilute in a drink as needed. When you do drink it, be warned that it's a pretty strong flavor! Wild oregano is also available in capsules to take orally.

Rosemary

Fights infection, reduces inflammation, is an antioxidant, and has a nice flavor.

Symphytum officinale

Also called comfrey, contains allantoin - a chemical which encourages bone, cartilage and muscle cells to grow. This explains why comfrey is called 'knitbone' by traditional healers, helping to heal wounds and injuries of all kinds.

Turmeric

This ancient herb from India is a potent antioxidant, anti-inflammatory, and antibiotic that is getting a lot of attention lately in research. Here are some more specific benefits against tumors and cancers[15]:

- Inhibit the proliferation of tumor cells
- Inhibit the transformation of cells from normal to tumor
- Help your body destroy mutated cancer cells so they cannot spread throughout your body

 www.wolfewellness.co

- Inhibit the synthesis of a protein thought to be instrumental in tumor formation
- Prevent the development of additional blood supply necessary for cancer cell growth
- Help ease discomfort in joints and muscles
- Enhance detoxification
- Improve gut health and digestion[16]

Also useful against these conditions:

- Cystic fibrosis
- Type 2 diabetes
- Crohn's disease
- Psoriasis
- Rheumatoid arthritis
- Cataracts
- Gallstones
- Muscle regeneration
- Inflammatory bowel disease
- Obesity: reduces the formation of fat tissue by suppressing the blood vessels needed to form it

Note that turmeric is much better for you when cooked rather than raw. The traditional Ayurvedic method is to quickly fry it, and other select spices, in gee for a minute before adding other foods to cook.

Because of its strong flavor, you might prefer to take this in a capsule. If so, here's a source that's ready to go: **Turmeric supplement**

Tusli (tea)

Try this for a nice, hot drink instead of black tea and coffee. This Ayurvedic herb has wonderful rejuvenating properties, may lower cortisol levels, has significant anti-inflammatory properties, and is mildly relaxing.

Tulsi Tea http://organicindia.mercola.com/Tulsi-Tea.aspx/?aid=CD426

Dietary nutrients

L-Arginine

This enhances the effectiveness of glutamine and fish oil by reducing inflammation. Supplement with 15-25 grams per day. Also helpful in the week before surgery. Take before food or at least 2 hours after. Can be taken along with other Amino Acid extracts (L-xyz).

Antioxidants

Consume lots of colorful fruit and veggies, especially dark leafy greens, cruciferous, citrus, berries and cherries. A green powder formula is a great way to supplement a diet lacking in these phytonutrients.

Glucosamine (sulfate) and Glycosamingens

These are well established in the literature for the repair of connective tissue. Aim for approximately 1500 milligrams daily

L-Glutamine

This simple yet powerful immune enhancing supplement is essential to speed your recovery. It also decreases inflammation, reduces dependency on narcotics, and improves liver function. It further enhances fish oil by reducing muscle wasting. A major use for high-dose glutamine would be to repair gastrointestinal injury. However, even though this is helpful in the short-term (1-2 months) for the above reasons, unless you lead a vigorously physical lifestyle to burn off the glutamine, then avoid long-term use in high doses. Take only on an empty stomach (20 minutes before food or at least 2 hours after). Can be taken along with other Amino Acid extracts (L-xyz).

L-Carnitine

One of the problems with avoiding red meat is lack of L-carnitine. Your body needs this amino acid for a healthy metabolism. It's especially good at powering up your muscles to burn fat. Bodybuilders consider it a "must" for staying ripped and strong. The problem is, as you get older, the amount of L-carnitine in your body starts to drop. To summarize, here's what this essential protein does for you:

- o *increases lean body mass while reducing body fat* ... an especially effective way to keep you lean and strong as you age.
- o increases bone mineral density and slows down bone loss
- o lowers cholesterol
- o decreases (sugar) cravings
- o balances blood sugar and blood pressure
- o For recovery purposes, regrowing lean muscle and bone is paramount. This is a must-have!

Take only on an empty stomach (20 minutes before food or at least 2 hours after). Can be taken along with other Amino Acid extracts (L-xyz).

MSM

Very potent nutrient to encourage healing and reduce swelling in the joints.

Rutin

Rutin is a flavonoid (others include hesperidin, quercetin, eriodictyl, and citron) and is essential for the absorption of vitamin C – so you should take it with your vitamin C to gain maximum benefit. It helps you recover because it decreases bruising and bleeding.

Bone, joint, & inflammation supplement

If you are looking to help your body rebuild from bone, joint, or unwanted inflammation, the combination formula called Triple Jointed could be a great benefit for you. It has already helped thousands of patients by uniting 5 powerful ingredients.

Greens supplements

A good wholefood supplement builds the blood, which in turn builds the body. They also alkalize the body, which helps it repair faster. Although there is an increasing number of companies jumping on this market, Dr. Young was the first micro-biologist to come out with a product. He continues to improve his product where others combine ingredients that look nice, but in fact subtract from the primary benefits, which are to alkalize the body and build the blood. So this formula is still the best quality and value available.

Combination post-op formulas

With this long list of items, you may be asking where to start. Although the following kit may not come to the high quality of the other individual recommendations, this does combine some of the useful supplements into a single package (multi-vitamin, enzymes, and homeopathic remedies for swelling/inflammation – *but not greens or other nutrients*). Note that although this is marketed for plastic surgery operations, it is still just as beneficial for most other recovery needs.

www.wolfewellness.co

Hormones

Serotonin

This naturally occurring chemical has a significant effect on mood and appetite. Most antidepressant medications prescribed today work by raising serotonin levels in the brain. Here are some good sources of this important hormone.

- o Bananas
- o Kiwis
- o Pineapples
- o Plantains
- o Plums
- o Tomatoes

Here are sources with moderate serotonin concentration:
- o Avocados
- o Black olives
- o Broccoli
- o Cantaloupe cauliflower
- o Dates
- o Eggplant
- ∩ Figs
- o Grapefruit
- o Honeydew melon
- o Spinach

Here is another not-so-obvious source:
- o Sunlight – yes plenty of bright sunlight during the day!
- o 5-HTP most potent over-the-counter source, but over 200 mg on an empty stomach can cause upset and should be avoided.

Melatonin

Known as the sleep hormone, it is also an important detox agent for your brain and an anti-inflammatory.

 www.wolfewellness.co

Enzymes

Enzymes are found in every cell of every living plant and animal, including humans. Enzymes are biocatalysts; which means that they either begin a reaction or cause a reaction to speed up. Without enzymes life would not exist.

Proteolytic

The proteolytic enzyme digests protein. Some examples of proteolytic enzymes are protease, serrapeptase, bromelain, and papain. Proteolytic enzymes are considered anti-inflammatory agents. Needed scar tissue will form and healing will take place significantly faster with the enzymes than without. You will also find that you heal without keloids (scare knots), surgical incisions will be less noticeable, joints will have less restrictions from post operative scar tissue and abdominal scar tissue that strangles the internal organs will not form. In central and Eastern Europe using systemic enzymes to speed healing and avoid scar tissue post operatively is standard practice with 40 years of application.

What is Fibrin?

Fibrin is the building block of connective tissue and as such, it is part of the body's repair mechanism. The deposition of fibrin is regulated by proteolytic enzymes. As age increases, fibrin production increases and enzymes output decreases thus, fibrin begins to grow in places it was not meant to be in abundance like our internal organs or across joints and muscles.

Can you stop taking the enzymes after they have eaten away at all the excess fibrin?

When you start to feel better, you may be tempted to stop taking the enzymes because they have done their job, however, if you do, the fibrin will grow back. It's important to continue taking the enzymes even after they have eaten away at the excess fibrin so that it will not return. At least continue for a few weeks, and then slowly decrease them to a level that works for you.

If we need fibrin as part of our repair mechanism, how do the enzymes know when to stop eating away at it?

The body marks the excess fibrin as exogenous protein so that our body knows that it is not needed. The enzymes will only attack exogenous proteins, leaving the endogenous proteins (those needed for repairs) to do their job.

What's the dosage?

Start taking the enzymes about 2 days after the surgery, provided you are not taking prescription blood thinners.

Co-enzyme Q10
  - Along with being very good for the heart in general, this has blood clotting effects similar to vitamin K. Also, CoQ10 produces impressive results during recovery from heart surgery. Note that **ubiquinol** is incredibly more effective than ubiquinone...by about 8 times. It's definitely worth it to get the one that works. CoQ10
    http://products.mercola.com/coq10-ubiquinol/?aid=CD426

Probiotics

It is vitally important that after taking any kind of antibiotics you should replenish the good bacteria in your gut. Here are a few reasons why:
  - It is important to maintain the good bacteria in your gut, which is essential for proper digestive function.
  - There are over 12 different strains of bacteria in your intestinal tract that are essential for your health.
  - These bacteria are a major part of your body's immune system.

www.wolfewellness.co

○ When selecting a probiotic, you want to get as many different strains and as many units as possible.

Detox

Before extolling the virtues of detoxing, be sensitive to the fact that your body is rebuilding itself after your operation (in small or large ways), so you may be too weak to detox just now and probably better off to save this step for when you're feeling stronger. That said, however, this will be an important step in your healing journey at some point, so you should still consider detoxing in the near future with a quality herbal cleanse formula – especially if your operation was required for a systemically caused problem (cancer, tumor, organ/system dysfunction), rather than a accident.

Think of your body like a car engine. If it's been running a long time and in rough conditions, it tends to get gunked up...so you take it to the shop and they clean the carburetor, replace the grimy spark plugs, dirty oil, and a host of other things. Well guess what – your body is a billion times more complex, has been subjected to multiple toxins/gunk for a long time, and will be able to repair itself far better if you clean it up. Of course, if your surgery involved any digestive organs, you'll want to consult your doctor for the best approach to this.

The best time of year to detox is in the spring when the weather warms up. The worst time is during winter when it's colder and your body wants to conserve itself.

A combination of Dr. Robert O. Young's greens and Dr. Jon Baron's detox makes an excellent start. An even stronger cleanse is the *Arise and Shine* package.

 www.wolfewellness.co

Juice

Juicing is your very best way to get most of your needed vitamins and other select food nutrients. While there are certainly many books on this subject, here are some basic principles to get you started:

- Use organic produce whenever possible. You'll be consuming more produce and you want to heal your body, so now is not the time to increase the toxic load with pesticide coated or GM foods.

- Focus 80% of your juicing on vegetables, and only 20% on fruits

- Don't mix fruit and vegetable juices in the same meal

- Drink about 50% equivalent of water with the juice

- Drink juices slowly and on an empty stomach (chew it a little or swish in the mouth) and at least 20 minutes before solid food

- Take some oil with the juice to help absorb the oil-based nutrients (olive, avocado, or krill are good). You can mix it in or just swallow a capsule...as you like.

- Listen to your body: if you react to a particular vegetable or blend (more than once), then use less/none of that

Don't have a juicer?

Here is one that is durable quality, easy to use and clean, and reasonably priced:
Fruit & Veg juicer
http://products.mercola.com/juicer/?aid=CD426

Morning alkalizing flush drink

This is an excellent way to start every day. I like to have this within 10 minutes of getting up.

- 1 pint filtered water (room temperature to very warm is better than cold)
- Some fresh-squeezed organic lemon (1/4 to 1 whole depending on size, juiciness, and preferences)
- 1/8 tsp unrefined salt (can be taken directly on the tongue and washed down; be mindful is your body is averse to salt)
- ½ tsp baking soda (made without aluminum). Best is pHour salts
- Sweeten to taste (Stevia recommended)
- Note that those who are particularly sensitive to sodium may want to reduce the salt and baking soda. Understand, however, that unrefined salt is much better for the body and less reactive on blood pressure than ordinary processed table salt. The pHour Salts are even better on your system (and would replace both the regular salt and baking soda in this recipe).

What to avoid

Foods to avoid

Face it, we do not live in a utopian paradise yet where everyone is looking out for our highest good. What does that mean for your food selection? Read the label of everything you intend to eat to ensure it does not contain anything in the list below.

Artificial sweeteners

Without listing them all and angering these big corporations, suffice it to say that no-one has yet produced an artificial sweetener that does not have

 www.wolfewellness.co

seriously dangerous side-effects. If you'd like more info on this, then read the book *Sweet Deception*.

http://products.mercola.com/sweet-deception/?aid=CD426

Caffeine

This drains your adrenal glands, vitamin B reserves, and choline. There are much better ways for a quick energy boost – and when you start implementing some of the changes in this book, you'll find you won't need quick boosts so often. A recent study showed that in some people, caffeine is not metabolized efficiently and therefore they can feel the effects long after consuming it.

Congestion causing foods

- o Dairy that is pasteurized (raw is less mucus forming)
- o Simple carbohydrates: refined wheat products, potatoes without skins, white rice

GM foods

Otherwise known as *genetically modified* foods. Sadly, one or two agricultural giants are trying to make an enormous profit by forcing the world to consume their patented seed products. GM foods come onto the market with negligible testing and therefore turn the mass population into their own giant testing ground. Do you really want to be the guinea pig for an outrageously unethical corporate profit grab? The other sad part is that after their infected Frankenstein seeds contaminate conventional and organic crops, it is very difficult to recover the natural genetic strain. So here's quick advice to avoid/minimize this effect on you and reduce their power:

- o Check the PLU codes of your produce (fruit/veg). It's a simple system:

- A 4-digit number means it's conventionally grown (pesticides, chemical fertilizers, etc)
- A 5-digit number starting with 8 means it's GM (avoid it!)
- A 5-digit number starting with 9 means it's organic (buy it)

o When foods have been processed in any way, manufacturers do not have to leave any hints whether it contains GM ingredients.

o When a grocery store packages the fruit themselves in their own packaging (like Cosco does) the PLU number only refers to that store's tracking and is no longer a relevant GM indicator.

o **Solution:** minimize processed foods (unless the ingredients are clearly labeled as organic), buy fresh and do your own cooking.

Hydrogenated oils

By now, most people are becoming aware of trans-fats. Manufacturers use them because these fats are cheap and have a long shelf-life. Your body on the other hand, has a serious problem with hydrogenated fats; in fact, they rank up near the top of most harmful foods you could possibly ingest.

MSG

Otherwise known as *monosodium glutamate*. This is another cheap trick that food manufacturers use to artificially enhance the flavor. MSG is a type of excito-toxin. That means that it is a toxic chemical that stimulates your sense of taste. It's toxic – avoid it.

Refined carbohydrates

These are the so-called *high glycemic carbs* that break down very quickly into simple sugars and therefore produce challenges similar to refined sugar. Some people can handle these better than others. If you exercise more, you may be able to burn off these calories, so it is a unique quantity for each individual. They include the following popular comfort foods:

- o White wheat – which is found in most breads, pastas, and pastries. Non-organic wheat in the USA is particularly toxic as it has been saturated with Glyphosate, which is a very toxic weed killer. Sourdough bread (organic) is healthier, and therefore generally ok for a small portion of the diet.

- o White rice

- o Potatoes – however, smaller potatoes eaten with their skins are acceptable in small quantities

The following grains are healthier, more alkalizing, and will help you reduce wheat-dominance in your diet:

- o Amaranth

- o Buckwheat

- o Kamut

- o Millet

- o Quinoa

- o Spelt

The way to make grains (and beans or nuts) healthier for you is to soak them at least 12 hours, then rinse, before cooking. If you'd like to go one step further, let them sit (damp, but not submersed) for another 24-48 hours to make them begin to sprout. Sprouted grains are nutritionally superior. Fermented grains are even better, but take much more effort, so I'm leaving that for you to research if you are inspired.

Refined sugar

Much has been discovered about the problems with refined (white) sugars:

- spikes the blood-sugar
- increases body fat
- paralyzes the immune system (the white blood cells)
- acidifies the body
- promotes chronic inflammation
- causes premature aging and skin spots
- interferes with sleep
- and many more

...that it should be obvious for someone who wants to heal fast and reclaim their health that they should avoid this. See the good substitutes in the Sweeteners section.

Along with sugar, beware of a common substitute: high fructose corn syrup. The problem with fructose is that when it's refined out of fruits (or corn or agave or any other starchy plant) it requires the liver to break it down – thus stressing your already over-worked liver. Dextrose/glucose is a healthier option as it gets converted to energy more efficiently.

When you have sugar cravings, it may not be the need for sugar, it might instead be a need for salt. As usual, each person needs to experiment by eating something salty to see if your sugar cravings go away. Best if the salt is unrefined.

Other ingestible things to avoid/minimize

Alcohol

This should be obvious, but it's got to be said.

Antibiotics

Although I can not legally tell you to avoid them, consider this about antibiotics:

- o They destroy much – and sometimes all – of your necessary digestive bacteria. Your gut bacteria is a major part of your immune system.

- o There are natural/herbal alternatives that are also effective, such as:

  - Colloidal silver, fresh garlic, and oil of oregano.

  - Note, however, that Colloidal silver can also reduce gut bacteria, so use as little as is needed and repopulate gut bacteria afterwards with probiotics and fermented foods.

Microwaved food

What's wrong with this? Well let's have a look:

- o From Dr. Lita Lee's book, *Health Effects of Microwave Radiation - Microwave Ovens*, and in the March and September 1991 issues of Earthletter: she stated that every microwave oven leaks electro-magnetic radiation, harms food, and converts substances cooked in it to dangerous organ-toxic and carcinogenic products. Further research summarized in this article reveal that microwave ovens are far more harmful than previously imagined.

o A study published in the November 2003 issue of The Journal of the Science of Food and Agriculture found that broccoli "zapped" in the microwave with a little water lost up to 97 percent of the beneficial antioxidant chemicals it contains. By comparison, steamed broccoli lost 11 percent or fewer of its antioxidants.

o When microwaving, carcinogenic toxins could be leached from your plastic and paper plates or covers and mix with your food.

o A 1991 lawsuit involving a woman (named Norma Levitt) who had hip surgery and died because the blood used in her blood transfusion was warmed in a microwave. Blood is routinely warmed before transfusions, but not by microwave. The microwave altered the blood and it killed the woman. Does it not therefore follow that this form of heating does, indeed, do 'something different' to the substances being heated? Is it not prudent to determine what that 'something different' might do?

o From the conclusions of the Swiss (Dr. Hans Ulrich Hertel), Russian (source: Atlantis Raising Educational Center in Portland, Oregon) and German scientific clinical studies, we can no longer ignore the microwave oven sitting in our kitchens. Based on this research, also note their conclusions:

- Continually eating food processed from a microwave oven causes long term - permanent - brain damage by "shorting out" electrical impulses in the brain [de-polarizing or de-magnetizing the brain tissue].

- The human body cannot metabolize [break down] the unknown by-products created in microwaved food.

- Male and female hormone production is shut down and/or altered by continually eating microwaved foods.

- The effects of microwaved food by-products are residual [long term, permanent] within the human body.

- Minerals, vitamins, and nutrients of all microwaved food is reduced or altered so that the human body gets little or no benefit, or the human body absorbs altered compounds that cannot be broken down.

- The minerals in vegetables are altered into cancerous free radicals when cooked in microwave ovens.

- Microwaved foods cause stomach and intestinal cancerous growths [tumors]. This may explain the rapidly increased rate of colon cancer in America.

- The prolonged eating of microwaved foods causes cancerous cells to increase in human blood.

    www.wolfewellness.co

- Continual ingestion of microwaved food causes immune system deficiencies through lymph gland and blood serum alterations.
- Eating microwaved food causes loss of memory, concentration, emotional instability, and a decrease of intelligence.

o Have you tossed out your microwave oven yet?

o **Solutions:**
  - After you throw out your microwave you can use a toaster oven as a replacement. It works well for most uses and is nearly as quick.
  - If you'd like something better than a toaster oven then Aroma's Turbo Oven is the solution: http://products.mercola.com/turbo-oven/?aid=CD426

Mercury

Mercury is a toxic, heavy metal and is becoming more prevalent. It's mainly a problem in large fish because they have longer lifetime to accumulate more mercury. Also, avoid fish from the Mediterranean Sea. If you need to purge your body of existing mercury, then Metal Magic is a powerful and easy forumula. http://www.clixgalore.com/PSale.aspx?BID=20558&AfID=189209&AdID=3233

Magnesium stereate

It's ironic the way respectable supplement manufacturers would use something toxic like this as a common processing agent in their tablets. This is similar to hydrogenated oil and used to help the particles of a tablet to flow through the machines and make it easier to produce the final tablet. However, it puts a strain on your immune system and reduces the effectiveness of whatever you are taking. Fortunately, there is a general trend to at least switch to vegetable based magnesium stereate...which is slightly better. In any case, avoid this as much as you can. It's usually listed as one of the *inactive* ingredients. Sprays and gel capsules won't have this.

Pain relievers: NSAIDS

Those innocent looking capsules are loaded with non-steroidal anti-inflammatory pain killers (NSAIDs), which is also the active ingredient in Benadryl. Sure, this unnatural chemical "cocktail" may get you through a sleepless night. But use it for a long time and you could pay a price.

- o They can break down intestinal tissue and may deplete folic acid and melatonin. Depletion of melatonin can cause sleep disturbances, problems with insulin regulation, and imbalances in immunity, and may also increase the risk of developing breast cancer.

- o Disturbances in your gastrointestinal tract and your natural flora can cause chronic inflammation, leading to a decrease in nutrient absorption, insulin resistance, and other metabolic disturbances.

- o Gastric erosions occur in almost half of individuals who take NSAIDs regularly. In the US, it has been estimated that about 16,500 deaths each year are related to NSAID use. NSAIDS have very well known side effects on intestinal and stomach linings.

- Acetaminophen (in Tylenol® PM and many cold and pain over-the-counter products) can be one of the most damaging drugs you can take! More than 30,000 cases per year of acetaminophen overdose are reported to the American Association of Poison Control Centers, and it is a leading cause of drug-induced liver failure in the US. There are some statistics showing even people taking modest dosages have damaged their livers.

- If you rely on these drugs to the exclusion of other methods – you may end up weakening your self-healing potential. Why risk it when there are such effective natural alternatives? There are an additional plethora of safer alternatives constantly becoming available.

Soy products

Although touted as a good protein source, here are some of the problems with this food.

- It is usually GM (genetically modified) unless it's labeled: Organic

- It contains large quantities of natural toxins or "antinutrients"

- It has one of the highest percentages contamination by pesticides of any of our foods

- It contains goitrogens - substances that depress thyroid function

- It is high in phytic acid, which can block the uptake of essential minerals - calcium, magnesium, copper, iron and especially zinc - in the intestinal tract

www.wolfewellness.co

There are many more facts about this, but this quick list gives you the general idea. Many people think that Asian's are benefited by this so why not others? Well the Asian diet uses only an average of a tablespoon per day and they mainly eat soy as a traditionally fermented product like miso or soy sauce. The fermentation process changes the chemistry to something much more beneficial.

In many pre-processed foods, soy is used as a cheap filler. So the bottom line is not to eat substantial quantities of this (like a meat substitute) and be sure it's always organic.

Smoking

Some people question why they need to give up smoking before/after surgery. The answer is simple: smoking and nicotine deprive the body of oxygen, and oxygen is essential not only to healing safely, but also to healing well.

It's important that you quit smoking at least two weeks before surgery and as many as eight weeks after surgery. This means no cigarettes or cigars, no nicotine patches or gum, and certainly no chewing tobacco/snuff.

Although this may seem difficult for one who's addicted, not smoking for several weeks may ultimately help you quit for life.

Ideally, you will then want to stay away from tobacco for the rest of your life.

- o **Solutions** - There are some effective programs to help.
  - ▪ EFT (Emotional Freedom Technique) – many people have successfully removed their psychological and physical cravings by using this

powerful energy technique. For more details, see the full section on EFT.

- Nicotine patches – many smokers use this simple, conventional method and make it work.
- Herbal/natural remedies – there are several good remedies that help to rapidly purge the body of all nicotine and thus remove the craving to maintain the nicotine level. That's another big topic!

Holistic remedies

These are nature's medicines. They have little or no side-effects, have been tried and tested (usually) for many more years than any conventional drug, have holistic/synergistic benefits, are (usually) non-addictive, and often produce a genuine feeling of well-being (not a dulled-drugged-stupor). They often work on the subtler, energetic level, which is being further understood every day. In a nutshell, everything is energy. Matter is simply vibrating at a slower frequency than things like electricity and light.

In 1994, the National Institutes of Health adopted a new term called a *Biofield* to describe the subtle energy field that extends outward from our bodies. This "vital energy" or "life force" is known under different names in different cultures such as *qi* (chi) in traditional Chinese medicine (TCM), *ki* in the Japanese Kampo system, and *doshas* in Ayurvedic medicine. Vital energy flows throughout the human body. Practitioners and therapists have been working with the body's Biofield for centuries to influence health.

Homeopathic

This form of medicine originated about 250 years ago. Therefore, we can consider it tried and true. The basic premise is that a miniscule treatment that produces similar effects as the ailment (that's the homeo part) will trigger your own body to correct the problem much faster and more effectively. Every homeopathic remedy has a strength number (like 6x, 12x, 30x, etc). This strength is the number of times it was potentiated, which increases its vital force. However, you may not always need the stronger dosage.

www.wolfewellness.co

Remedies are usually taken under the tongue (sublingually), topically in a cream base, or mixed in water. When taking topically, there's no need to rub or massage into the skin – simple contact of your skin (where it hurts) with the formula is fine. If you'd like to know more about homeopathy, then see this link for starters: http://en.citizendium.org/wiki/Homeopathy

Homeopathy will be even more effective if you get a customized formula from a qualified practitioner. You will need to conduct your own search to find a local therapist.

Arnica montana 30

Can be used topically and orally. Arnica Montana has been used for centuries to treat swelling, soreness and bruising. Derived from the dried roots of the arnica plant (part of the daisy family and sometimes called leopard's bane), is a highly respected ingredient in homeopathic medicine. Arnica has powerful anti-inflammatory, tissue healing, and antibacterial properties, and it is thought to stimulate white blood cells to facilitate healing and help eliminate excess fluid/bleeding from traumatized areas.

Many surgeons recommend taking three tablets three times per day, starting as many as two weeks before surgery and continuing 3x per day after surgery to help with the healing process. In fact, a study published last year in the Archives of Facial Plastic Surgery showed that those who took arnica had 24% less bruising after a facelift than those who took a placebo.

Although naturally derived, arnica should not be used on broken skin; when taken orally, the recommended dose should not be exceeded. Those with sensitive stomachs should use arnica with caution.

While there are different doses of homeopathic arnica available at health food stores and websites, such Arnica products are simply not strong enough to treat surgery patients. SinEcch has been proven to be the most effective dosage strength for reducing bruising and swelling after surgery

Aconite 200 or 30

Can be taken if there is substantial fear.

Calendula 30

Can be taken to promote healthy tissue, prevent infection, and speed healing.

Hypericum 30

Can be used topically and orally. Topically, place 10 drops in a cup of clean water. Use three-four times a day until the wound is healed.

Magnesium phosphoricum D6

Is a biochemic tissue salt found naturally occurring in the body. It is known as the 'homeopathic aspirin' due to its unique pain killing and curative properties and is also an effective muscle relaxant, preventing and treating spasms and cramps and promoting relaxation.

Matricaria recutita C6

Is known for its soothing, anti-inflammatory and pain relieving properties.

Phosporus 30

Can be taken after anesthetic to remove poison

SinEcch™ strong combination formula

Pronounced [sin' ekk] - is a medicine prepared in accord with the FDA's regulations for Homeopathic preparations. Made from Arnica Montana, SinEcch™ is the only Arnica Montana dosage regimen that is clinically proven to significantly reduce bruising and swelling after surgery.

SINECCH™ has been safely used for hundreds of thousands of surgeries over the past 10 years and has become an increasingly common treatment in many other healing regimes. Physicians and patients alike find that using SINECCH™ helps speed the post-operative recovery process, reducing uncomfortable swelling and bruising and often post-operative pain, as well.

By using SinEcch right before and after a surgery, a patient is able to minimize bruising and swelling, have less post-operative pain and discomfort, accelerate the healing process, and shorten recovery time. Designed specifically for plastic surgery patients, SinEcch is also used for recovery from a wide range of non-cosmetic, general surgeries and procedures and for the treatment of various kinds of traumatic injuries. SinEcch can also help reduce the swelling of the face and gums and the bruising of gums and skin that sometimes occur after oral surgeries including root canal, dental implant, and wisdom tooth removal.

SinEcch   http://www.makemeheal.com/mmh/product.do?id=10369

Bach flower remedies

The Bach Flower Remedies® are dilutions of a very small amount flower material in a 50:50 solution of water and brandy. Because the remedies are extremely dilute they do not have a characteristic scent or taste of the plant. As such, they are a safe and natural method of healing. They gently restore the balance between mind and body by casting out negative emotions, such as, fear, worry, hatred and indecision which interfere with the equilibrium of the being as a whole. The Bach Flower Remedies® allow peace and happiness to return to the sufferer so that the body is free to heal itself. Therefore, take a careful look at these remedies because leaving negative emotions to simmer will defeat all your other efforts to heal.

Dr. Edward Bach was a British Physician and homeopath, in the 1930s, who began to see disease as an end product; a final stage; a physical manifestation of unhappiness, fear and worry. He therefore, began to look to nature to find healing flowers. Over a period of years Dr. Bach found 38 healing flowers and plants that with the right preparation became the 38 Bach Flower Remedies®. These Remedies are enough to remove all negative emotional problems.

Although Bach flower remedies often are associated with homeopathy, the remedies are distinct from homeopathy in that they do not follow fundamental homeopathic precepts such as the *law of similars* or the assumption that curative powers are enhanced by diluting and shaking (succussion).

There is no risk in taking the wrong flower remedy because it simply will not do what you want. In other words, it will not produce any unwanted side-effects (the way many allopathic drugs might).

www.wolfewellness.co

The best known flower remedy is the Rescue Remedy combination, which contains an equal amount each of Rock Rose, Impatiens, Clematis, Star of Bethlehem, and Cherry Plum essences. The product is aimed at treating stress, anxiety, and panic attacks, especially in emergencies.

It's not difficult to survey the 38 remedies and decide which ones you feel you need. However, a little education will make this treatment much more effective. So you may wish to read a booklet, attend a workshop, or visit a practitioner.

www.wolfewellness.co

Physical & topical remedies

This section covers external things that you can do to enhance and speed the healing process.

Hot/cold therapy

Important to note here is that cold reduces inflammation and strengthens the vascular system while challenging the immune system a little bit. If you have any kind of cold/flu or other contraindicated conditions, then start slow and go easy on the cold treatments until you're body is stronger.

With a compress

Specialized cold and hot compresses can effectively provide both cold and hot therapy to swollen and bruised areas. As surgery can cause post-operative swelling and bruising, cold and hot therapy is needed to help reduce these symptoms. Cold therapy is very effective for reducing the initial swelling, relieving sensations of pain, and accelerating the healing process for the first few days after surgery. To cool your wound this way, simply place an ice-pack (a soft, reusable pack is best) for about 20 minutes – no longer or you'll slow circulation too much and inhibit healing. You can do this as many as 10x/day as needed. If possible, it also helps to elevate your wound.

Hot therapy (only after about 3-5 days when initial swelling has gone down) helps break down and disintegrate bruising discolorations and provides moisture or dry heat to areas of discomfort.

www.wolfewellness.co

In the shower

Since blood circulation is what helps your body repair itself faster, this therapy should become a part of your daily routine. By alternating hot and cold in certain intervals, it drives the blood to the extremities, then to your core, and then back again – over and over. It's almost as good at improving your circulation as exercising. When it's ok for you to take a shower, here's what you do:

1. Take your normal wash with soap in warm water (not hot or cold)
2. Turn the faucet to a warmer temperature and get the heat over as much as your body as possible for about 20-30 seconds.
3. Turn the faucet to a cool temperature and get the coolness over as much as your body as possible for about 30-60 seconds.
4. Repeat steps 2 and 3 up to 6 times.
5. Always finish with cold to lock in the warm blood.
6. As you get used to this treatment, increase the difference in the temperatures until your standing under the hottest and coldest water you can.
7. If you can make to a Korean or Russian bath spa, then they'll have hot and cold pools waiting for you!

Note – this therapy makes it even more important to have a chlorine filter on your shower. **Shower Filter**.
http://products.mercola.com/shower-filter-pure-clear/?aid=CD426
Note – Slavic, Germanic, and other cultures have benefited from hot/cold baths for centuries and this type of bath house is common in most of their cities.

Infrared & laser light therapy

Low-level laser therapy is the application of red and near-infrared light over injuries or wounds to improve soft tissue healing and relieve both acute and chronic pain. Low-level therapy uses cold (subthermal) laser light energy to direct bio-stimulative light energy to the body's cells without injuring or damaging them in any way. The therapy is precise and accurate; and offers safe and effective treatment for a wide variety of conditions.

When low level laser light waves penetrate deeply into the skin, they optimize the immune responses of our blood. This has both anti-inflammatory and immunosuppressive effects. It is a scientific fact that light transmitted to the blood in this way has positive effective throughout the whole body, supplying vital oxygen and energy to every cell. In summary, here is what they can do for your healing process:

- Relieve acute and chronic pain
- Increase the speed, quality and tensile strength of tissue repair
- Increase blood supply
- Stimulate the immune system
- Stimulate nerve function
- Develop collagen and muscle tissue
- Help generate new and healthy cells and tissue
- Promote faster wound healing and clot formation
- Reduce inflammation

Infrared light relieves pain, stiffness, and spasm -- and enhances your blood circulation. You get this naturally with sunlight. You can also benefit from this from the following devices:

- Infrared plus red light panels: https://redtherapy.co/?rfsn=7906775.8a8c7c&utm_source=refersion&utm_medium=affiliate&utm_campaign=7906775.8a8c7c
- Infrared heating lamp: most large, conventional hardware stores have these.

Hyperbaric Oxygen Therapy (HBOT)

Hyperbaric oxygen therapy was first used in the U.S. in the early 20th century.

HBOT helps wound healing by bringing oxygen-rich plasma to tissue starved for oxygen. Wound injuries damage the body's blood vessels, which release fluid that leaks into the tissues and causes swelling. This swelling deprives the damaged cells of oxygen, and tissue starts to die.

HBOT offers a safe, natural, and efficient medical therapy for non-healing incision wounds. Since HBOT addresses wound healing at a deep cellular level, it can be used to address surgical wounds that are struggling to heal properly.

Note that HBOT is not for everyone. It shouldn't be used by people who have had a recent ear surgery or injury, a cold or fever, or certain types of lung disease.

Natural wound spray

Among recent scientific healing breakthroughs is a natural spray that makes your skin heal much faster – and is especially good with burns because it treats the skin itself.

Very simple to use and inexpensive, you will quickly feel the results. Find out more from the link below: Wound Spray   http://www.myonlineshoppingcart.com/app/?af=959660

Compression garments

Compression under-clothes can be helpful in supporting the part of your body that was weakened by the surgery. This is a discretionary choice as your individual needs will be unique to your operation, your preferences, and your lifestyle.

Compression Garments   http://makemeheal.directtrack.com/z/272/CD790

Exercises

Exercise is essential to good health. It should go without saying, but there are still those – including most physicians – who fail to understand this. What exercises you do and how soon into your recovery will vary considerably depending on your surgery. Take care with any exercise, start slowly, and consult your doctor beforehand if you're not sure whether something is appropriate for you. This list is designed with recovery in mind. These are some basic, gentle, and rejuvenating exercises that can really help you heal faster and more completely.

Exercise is an underappreciated tool to treat disease. So, why exercise?

- Belly fat is a huge source of inflammation; it puts out inflammatory compounds like IL-6 and TNF-alpha
- Stimulate blood-flow to assist with cell repair
- Stimulate lymphatic circulation/drainage to speed detoxing and well-being

www.wolfewellness.co

- Circulate all those wonderful herbs/supplements/nutrients from your dietary regime throughout your body
- Reduce high blood pressure (hypertension)
- Improve the immune system
- Boost natural life force energy known as Chi
- Some of these exercises go even further towards your healing by targeting and strengthening weakened areas

If you get this eBook before your surgery, then you are in an ideal position to strengthen those areas that will be affected by the operation. This is *very significant* because the stronger you make the affected areas, the faster and more comfortably they will recover.

Walking

This most basic exercise is something you should do as soon as you're able – even if only a little at first. Work up to at least 30 minutes/day. Also, it's a nice way to settle a meal.

Elephant Swing

This is an excellent exercise you could start even when you're barely able to walk.

Benefits:
- Excellent starter exercise, very gentle
- Releases tension in the entire body and soothes the emotional state – also a good preparation for sleep or to shake off bed stiffness in the morning
- Gives your body a gentle toning
- Circulates lymphatic fluid and blood
- Rejuvenates your eyes too

 www.wolfewellness.co

How to do it:

1. Place your feet about shoulder-width apart and drop your hands loosely to the sides.

2. Turn your body at the waist as far to one side as it will comfortably go and then gently swing back to the other side as far as it will go. Initiate the turn from your belly button, rather than from your head or shoulders.

3. Allow your arms to swing freely during this rotation. Move your head in line with your shoulders... don't keep your head stationary.

4. Either shift your weight from one foot to the other as you swing from side to side or keep them equal, depending how your body feels. To shift weight, allow the trailing heel to lift up from the ground a little (so on a swing to the left, the right heel would lift).

5. Your eyes could be halfway open and relaxed – a little dreamy. You can also try closing them in the beginning. Keep them at the same horizontal level – don't look up/down. During the swing, relax your eyes and facial muscle without attempting to see any object. If you feel a little dizzy, remember to not fixate the eyes on any single object, but just let them scan across all passing objects as they follow your swinging.

6. Ideally, do this exercise outside (barefoot in the sun) or in front of a big window with a distant view.

7. For added benefit, take some deep sighs during this exercise, and say a big, long "aaahhhhhh." This will aid further relaxing affect and release tense energy from the liver.

 www.wolfewellness.co

8. Do this swing slowly (about 1.5 seconds to swing in one direction). Swing about 30 seconds to begin, then work up to 5 minutes which is about 100 swings (back-and-forth equals 1 swing). From 1-60 swings, your body relaxes; from 60-100 you fully release nerves and muscles. You can do this exercise 3-4 times/day.

9. After swinging, just sit or lie down peacefully and you will enjoy the feeling of chi energy awakening in your body.

Links to videos:

- This one has a qigong (pronounced chi-gong) background: https://www.youtube.com/watch?v=98ODPvKrGlg
- This one shows alternating weight and brings in other activities to improve eyesight as well: https://www.youtube.com/watch?v=7agJ9lxSHEw

Breathing

When breath volume, rate and attention level are all altered, dramatic physiological, and even emotional, changes can occur. As it turns out, unknown to science until very recently, the action of the lungs, diaphragm and thorax are a primary pump for the lymph fluid, a lymph heart.

The act of relaxed, full breathing moves the function of the autonomic nervous system towards balance or homeostasis.

Empirical science, the scientific method of all original cultures, is based on trial and error. That which has value is kept and employed. That which is found to have little or no value is dropped. In the empirical approach, that which is kept, is "tried and true". Empirically breath practice is "tried and true".

Individuals who are well are able to remain well; they adapt to greater stress and have greater endurance when they keep breath practice in their daily self-care routine. Inspiration is the rush that one feels when over taken by spiritual energy, it is the force that impels one forward into life, and it is the divine influence that brings forth creativity and vitality.

Notice your own breathing. Isn't each breath very shallow?

If you note carefully you will probably realize that you are utilizing one quarter or less, of your lung capacity.

Because most modern people are addicted to excessive thinking and busyness, reaching a state of authentic relaxation is a challenge. Many of us are locked into worry, hurry, overwork, and compulsive behaviors and so the mind is very difficult to quite.

The beauty of these progressive relaxation processes is their simplicity and their ability to allow the mind to have an easy focus. When the attention wanders off of the process one need only return to the breath and the sequence of awareness points.

Full Chest and Abdominal Breathing
- This method is simply a deepening of the breath. Take slow, deep, rhythmic breaths through the nose. When the diaphragm drops down, the abdomen is expanded allowing the air to rush into the vacuum created in the lungs.

- Then the chest cavity is expanded, allowing the lungs to fill completely. This is followed by a slow, even exhalation which empties the lungs completely.

- This simple breath practice done slowly and fully, with intention, concentration and relaxation activates all of the primary benefits of therapeutic breath practice.

www.wolfewellness.co

- In both Qigong and Pranayama, you can learn more advanced methods and sometimes the breath is an further retained for additional benefit.

Simple method that initiates the relaxation response.
- Begin by taking slow deep breaths. Repeat these messages to yourself.
- "My hands and arms are heavy and warm" (5 times).
- "My feet and legs are heavy and warm" (5 times).
- "My abdomen is warm and comfortable" (5 times).
- "My breathing is deep and even" (10 times).
- "My heartbeat is calm and regular" (10 times). "My forehead is cool" (5 times).
- "When I open my eyes, I will remain relaxed and refreshed" (3 times).

A more vigorous form of breathing, when you feel strong enough, has been popularized by Wim Hof and his method. This is a very powerful way to build back stronger!

https://www.youtube.com/watch?v=nzCaZQqAs9I

Chi Gung (Qigong)

Pronounced "chee gong," while this practice is about 5,000 years old and there are today numerous courses/teachers available, I have found Spring Forest Qigong to be the easiest to learn and the one most focused on healing injuries and illness.

Everything in the universe is a form of energy: your mind, your spirit (consciousness), and even your body. All sicknesses of your body, mind, or spirit are caused by energy blockages. Spring Forest Qigong helps you remove those blockages and transform that energy.

The goal of Spring Forest Qigong is to enhance the quality of your life by teaching you ways to open your energy channels and maintain balance. When you remove the imbalance, you remove the pain, the problem, and the cause of the problem.

A great side-benefit of this practice is that you can really develop a new and unique feeling of this tangible energy as it makes your body, mind, and spirit much stronger and vigorous. This is why it is the method that millions of people use to stay strong and healthy as they get older so they can continue living an active, positive, and long life.

Qigong is the grandfather of Chinese medicine, including Tai-Chi, acupuncture, and Shiatsu. Some say it is the basis for Reiki and similar practices. But only in the past few decades has its medical nature become widespread in China and now known to the rest of the world. In a PBS documentary, Dr. Wang Chong Xing from the Shanghai Institute of Hypertension said that after 30 years of study,

"We think Qigong can cure every kind of disease, some responding better than others."

An easy, affordable, and effective way to learn this is from the **Qigong DVD** .
http://www.1shoppingcart.com/app/?af=976414

Laughter as healing

Laughter has a real beneficial effect on your physical health, which has been verified by ample research. In one study, subjects were observed as they watched both serious movies and comedies. During the comedies, their arteries dilated and their blood pressure dropped, suggesting that laughter can in fact be a powerful medicine indeed.

www.wolfewellness.co

These are the benefits shown from this research:

- Blood flow was significantly reduced (by about 35 percent) in 14 of the 20 volunteers who saw the stressful film
- Blood flow significantly increased (by 22 percent) in 19 of the 20 volunteers after watching the funny movie
- The improvement in blood flow experienced by most all participants after laughter was equal to the improvements seen after a 15- or 30-minute workout!

To summarize the benefits from other research, laughter:

- Causes your body to release beneficial chemicals called endorphins, natural "pain killers" that contribute to your sense of well-being and may counteract the effects of stress hormones and cause blood vessels to dilate.
- Relaxes and reduces muscle tension
- Lowers production of stress hormones
- Improves/strengthens your immune system
- Reduces blood pressure
- Clears your lungs by dislodging mucous plugs
- Increases the production of salivary immunoglobulin A, which defends against infectious organisms that enter through your respiratory tract
- Aerobic effects that increase your body's ability to utilize oxygen
- Provides a rapid ability to disregard aches and pains or to perceive them as less severe
- Increases your intellectual performance and boosts information retention

 www.wolfewellness.co

- Just anticipating laughter can increase your endorphin levels, whereas laughing may help boost your immune system and reduce inflammation in your body

- Helps you to stay positive and happy. Happy people live longer, are healthier, are more successful, enjoy more fulfilling relationships, earn more money, and are liked and respected more

To improve your state of mind and laugh more – besides renting a stack of comedies – see the tools in the sections: EFT, Sedona, and Chi Gung.

Egoscue method

The Egoscue Method is a widely acclaimed Postural Therapy program based on a series of stretches and gentle exercises designed to restore full, natural function to muscles and joints. It is a unique and very effective program designed to treat musculoskeletal pain *without* drugs, surgery, or manipulation. This means that if your surgery (or any current condition) resulted from any repetitive injury syndrome or postural problem, then this is very important for you to prevent further damage and perhaps achieve complete recovery.

You can get the generic serious of these stretches and gentle exercises from his books or visit their clinics to receive exercises specifically designed for each client. This process strengthens specific muscles and brings the body back to its proper alignment and functioning the way it was designed—pain free.

Although this method is headquartered in San Diego, CA, they have practitioners throughout the USA, Mexico, and Japan. If none of these locations work for you, then you may be interested in trying their live video conferencing.

Yoga stretching

This ancient method will rejuvenate, strengthen, tone, and flex your body in many wonderful and enjoyable ways. This is best done with a live teacher experienced in recovery. Use your discretion and instructor's advice as to which type of yoga, how to much you should practice, and which movements you can perform.

There are local instructors virtually everywhere and it's hard to find a bad one!

Mini-trampoline - rebounding

This exercise is better left until you're past the initial, fragile stages of recuperation because it puts a bit more strain on the body. However, don't let that stop you when you're strong enough because it's widely proven to be one of the best exercises for you entire body. To understand this, just realize that when you bounce, every single cell in your body suddenly gets exercise: they all have to resist the change in direction. Also, this is a cushioned bounce, so is more gentle than just jumping on the ground (as with a jump-rope, for example). More than any other exercise, rebounding circulates your lymphatic system.

There is ample research and testimonies about this exercise, so you could easily spend a few hours if you'd like to study this topic further. Rebounder
http://www.phmiracleliving.com/p-350-half-fold-rebounder.aspx?affiliateid=10152

Visualize your exercises

Why? Because when you imagine that you are doing something, your nerves, your cells, your muscles, your brain - everything that is part of you - gets the message and responds accordingly.

- Even if you're stuck in bed, you can still train in your imagination. And doing so will have a healing effect beyond what you can fathom.

- Throughout history, there have been stories of strongmen who rose from their deathbeds - from a weak, sickly state of ill health - and became powerful.

- They didn't just survive the tough time. They thrived.

- The key is understanding that success is a combination of physical practice and mental practice. He who does both rises to the greatest heights of achievement. In fact, in any endeavor on the face of the earth, if you were to ask the question "How much of success is mental" to those at the top, the most common reply would be "Most of it. Ninety percent or more."

Exercise combo treatment

When you realize that your body thrives on the following elements:

- **Sun** – gives the best vitamin D, infrared, serotonin, and positive emotional boost

- **Earth** – grounds out static electricity and recharges subtle energies

- **Sweat** – flushes toxins and circulates all those wonderful herbs/supplements/nutrients from your dietary regime

Then you can appreciate that the combination of doing your exercises in a bathing suit, under the mid-day sun, and barefoot on the earth (sand/dirt is slightly better than grass) is a fantastic treatment! It's ironic how the most basic lifestyle of our species for the last 2 million or so years is so beneficial...back to basics indeed.

Massage

Along with exercise, massage is very helpful to relieve pain, break up fibrosis, prevent adhesions, relieve swelling, and improve circulation. When skin is touched, rubbed, or massaged, the local immune cells increase their activity. Of course, it can also go far beyond that as you will soon see.

Self-massage on outer scar tissue

From the previous sections you can understand that your hands have great healing energy. That's how "laying-on of hands" works. After your operation heals enough (and you can confirm the best time with your surgeon), you can begin rubbing the scar area – or around it. This is incredibly helpful to stimulate healing. Gently at first, rubbing along the scar and outside it is very good. Do this at least twice a day (especially before bed) for 5-20 minutes. Using a combination of the oils below is even better.

Formula for your own homemade post-op massage oil (don't worry about getting the proportions exact):

- Castor oil   -   20%
- Lavender oil -   20%
- Aloe vera   -   15%
- Shea oil   -   10%
- Honey   -   10%   (should be organic, unfiltered, and unheated)
- Vitamin E   -   10%
- Bee propolis -   5%

www.wolfewellness.co

- Tea tree oil   -   5%
- Vitamin D oil -   5%

Lymphatic

The lymphatic system has no pump like the heart to circulate it, so it depends on certain physical stimuli. This means specific exercises or massage. Lymphatic massage can make you feel wonderful if these fluids are congested.

You will need to conduct your own search for local practitioners.

Cranio-sacral therapy

A craniosacral therapy session involves the therapist placing their hands on the patient, which allows them to tune into what they call the craniosacral system. This technique relieves restrictions of nerve passages, optimizes the movement of cerebrospinal fluid through the spinal cord, and can even restore misaligned bones to their proper position. Craniosacral therapists use the therapy to treat mental stress, neck and back pain,migraines, TMJ Syndrome, and for chronic pain conditions such as fibromyalgia. In some European countries, there is always a craniosacral therapist at the birth of every child to gently realign the infants skull after the trauma of the birth canal. In addition, and definitely not the least of the benefits, this massage therapy can have dramatic results in releasing old, negative, pent-up emotions.

You will need to conduct your own search for local practitioners.

Upper Cervical Chiropractic

This gentle, non-invasive technique was developed more than forty years ago to create a radical new way of healing that can help restore body balance and perfect health. The focus of the NUCCA work is the relationship between the upper cervical spine (neck) and its influence on the central nervous system and brain stem function. It is this relationship that affects every aspect of human function from the feeling sensations in your fingers to regulating hormones, controlling movement, and providing the ability to hear, see, think, and breathe.

There are many ways this critical head/neck area can become misaligned; a fall, an accident, a bump on the head, bad sleeping habits or poor posture. Misalignment can even occur during the birth process. Forceps used as a birthing aid, or a simple twist of the head during delivery can bring on misalignment! Any type of misalignment, regardless of how it occurred, restricts or distorts brain to body messages in this critical area at the top of the neck. Left unchecked this misalignment can cause pain and symptoms to develop and increase during one's lifetime.

Here's one site where you can search for local practitioners. http://www.nucca.org/find_doctor.php

Acupuncture and acupressure

Acupuncture is based on the precepts of traditional Chinese Medicine that says the body and mind are inextricably linked; that vital energy, or chi (also spelled qi), regulates a person's spiritual, emotional, mental and physical health; that each of us is a delicate balance of opposing and inseparable forces called yin and yang -- and when that balance is disrupted, vital energy becomes blocked or weakened. When our qi (energy) is at optimal levels and flowing smoothly, we're ready to take on the world. Spiritually, emotionally, mentally and physically we're strong, healthy and energized.

If the needles scar you, then an acupressure may be your thing. This could also include massage that helps your chi flow better.

Both can be great for immediate and long-term pain relief.

If you'd like to try acupressure on yourself here's a free guide online: http://arthritis.about.com/gi/dynamic/offsite.htm?zi=1/XJ /Ya&sdn=arthritis&cdn=health&tm=194&f=10&tt=14&bt= 1&bts=1&zu=http://www.geocities.com/jrh_iii/acupressur e/acupoints.html

You will need to conduct your own search for local practitioners.

Environmental hazards to avoid

Plastics

This pervasive material is so embedded in our food routines that avoiding it may seem difficult. Most plastics leach toxic dioxins into your food...especially at higher temperatures like your car on a warm day or the microwave. This is a known cause of cancer. Also, when plastic containers are washed in hot water and detergent, the chemical composites break down and begin leaching at any temperature.

Solutions:
- Store leftovers in glass containers
- Keep your drinking water in a stainless steel or glass container (the glass VOSS bottles of water make excellent reusable containers because their lid doesn't wear out like metal lids)
- Especially avoid storing hot/oily foods – such as coffee cups or take-away meals – in Styrofoam (foamed polystyrene) because it immediately leaches toxic benzene and other chemicals into the food.

Constipation

Ok, so this is not strictly an environmental hazard, but this *inner* environment issue will work against your recovery. If you've begun following the dietary recommendations in this eBook, then this problem ought to clear up within a few weeks and stay away effortlessly. In the short term, however (now), it is critical to eliminate toxins from your bowel at least every day. If you don't believe that, then you can get convinced here:

Helpful tips:

- One possible cause of this condition is a lack of fiber-rich foods...so eat more of them. Vegetables are phenomenal sources of fiber (raw is best). See the dietary sections above for those details.

- For added fiber to help normalize your stool, try organic flaxseeds. Just grind the seeds in a coffee grinder, then add a tablespoon or two to your food. If you buy pre-ground seeds, then keep them in an airtight container in the refrigerator. Drink more liquids whilst taking this and monitor results to avoid over-doing.

- The simplest home remedy is prune juice.

- Lesser known, but probably the most healthy approach would be to take magnesium carbonate or magnesium oxide to break up this stuck matter.

- Try squatting. This is the best, natural position to help expel stool from your colon and reduce your risk of hemorrhoids, and it's still the way many people around the world go to the bathroom. In your home, you can get many of the same benefits by placing a stool near your toilet to raise your knees, purchasing a special squatting device to modify your toilet, or simply squatting on your own toilet.

- You can also try organic psyllium, which you can use nearly every day. Psyllium is unique because it's an adaptogenic fiber, which means it will help soften your stool if you're constipated, or reduce frequency of your bowel movements if you have loose stools.

- Exercise regularly. This helps stimulate circulation and intestinal function, causing your bowels to move properly. A simple 10-minute walk is very helpful; additionally, if you bring up each knee with each step for a short while, this will further stimulate the digestive tract.

www.wolfewellness.co

- Enzymes can also come to the rescue here. See the supplement sections above for those details.
- Take a high-quality probiotic. They are also useful in fighting IBS, which can contribute to constipation.

- Aloe vera is also an excellent way to sooth and speed up your bowel movements.
- Get checked for hypothyroidism, especially if you're a woman over 40. Constipation is one of the hidden symptoms of hypothyroidism.
- Avoid commercial (and stimulant) laxatives. Commercial laxatives are too harsh and may contain unwanted toxic additives. One of the biggest risks of stimulant laxatives is that your body can become dependent on them for normal bowel function. When you stop using them, it takes a long time for the activity of your bowel to be restored.
- This is true even of senna, cassia laxatives, and casgara sagrada, which are frequently marketed as natural. However, these natural remedies are good for 1-3 uses to "uncork" the problem.
- The commercial and these 2 herbal laxatives, when used for a period of weeks or months, may even decrease your colon's natural ability to contract, which will worsen constipation. Further, overuse of laxatives can damage nerves, muscles and tissues of your large intestine.
- So if you absolutely must use a laxative, make sure it is only for a very short-term period. And remember that laxatives do absolutely nothing to address the underlying causes of your constipation. But fortunately the natural tips in the above section do.

www.wolfewellness.co

Geopathic stress

This is electro-magnetic stress that naturally occurs at any particular point on our planet's surface. It can come from underground streams, veins of electrically charged metal and even deeper things in the Earth. When you pass through these areas, you are not consciously aware (most people, most of the time) and they have little affect. However, if you stay on them for extended periods (sleeping on a bed, sitting at table/desk), then their cumulative effects will drain your body of vital energy and make health and recovery that much harder. It is even possible that this negative energy has weakened your body to the point that it required surgery to repair the problem. Now think about going home and lying down on that very same thing that caused the problem...do you think your recovery will come quickly? Not as likely. Do take this seriously.

Helpful tips:
- **Move your bed** – If you have trouble sleeping despite trying several of my guidelines for a good night's sleep (in the sleep section of this eBook), then try moving your bed several feet to one side or the other, or to the opposite side of the room so see if it makes a difference. If you find yourself sleeping more soundly in another area of your bedroom, or even in another room of your house, it may be well worth it to stick with it. It's quite likely your body is responding to unseen energy disturbances. Checking this for chairs/couches will be more difficult because most people can't consciously feel a difference.

- **Dowsing** – you would need to hire a trained dowser to come to your house and determine which places in your house have geopathic stress. They would then advice you as to more positive locations to move the furniture that you spend the most time in. https://www.youtube.com/watch?v=LueWGX5arYY

- **Counter-balancing frequency** – this is where you keep your body charged with healthy frequencies that are much stronger than the unhealthy ones coming up from the ground. There are many devices that purport to do just this, so consult an expert for latest and greatest tech.

Chemically treated furnishings & clothes

Toxins from flame-retardant items are constantly out-gassing. This means the chemical causing their flame resistance is leaking into the air...that you are breathing. You should minimize this exposure by examining your clothes, bed, sheets, furniture, and anything else near you to find out if it's flame resistant (and then replace them). While you should do what you can to prevent the house and everything else burning down, the cost to your body that has to absorb these toxins is equally devastating.

Manufactured negative energies

This topic is slowly gaining recognition as it also has serious impacts on your body's recovery. For instance, if you are being bombarded with strong EMFs and wireless frequencies, it's possible they already contributed to weakening your body in a way that could have led to the very problem you are recovering from. In any case, you'll want to minimize this impact to speed your recovery.

EMFs (electro-magnetic frequencies)

An EMF is an invisible zone of energy that surrounds <u>all electrical devices and wiring</u>. Electrical appliances – TVs, blenders, washers, microwaves, etc all generate harmful EMFs while they operate.

At one time it was believed that low-level magnetic fields were not harmful, but scientists now agree that EMFs are indeed hazardous to human health. They are now considered "probable carcinogens," and have been linked to cases of childhood leukemia, lymphoma and other health conditions. The exact mechanism by which exposure leads to cancer has not been established. But one potential mechanism may be due to EMFs ability to alter the expression of certain genes; turning them on and off at inappropriate times, which may cause them to initiate cell proliferation.

Additionally, the BioInitiative Report, (http://www.bioinitiative.org/) published August 31, 2007 by an international working group of scientists, researchers and public health policy professionals, documents serious scientific concerns about the radiation emitted from power lines, cell phones, and many other sources of exposure to radiofrequencies and electromagnetic fields in daily life.

It concludes that the existing standards for public safety are completely inadequate to protect your health. The report includes studies showing evidence that electromagnetic fields can:

- Affect gene and protein expression (Transcriptomic and Proteomic Research)
- Have genotoxic effects – RFR and EMF DNA damage
- Induce stress response (Stress Proteins)
- Affect immune function
- Affect Neurology and behavior
- Cause childhood cancers (Leukemia)
- Cause Alzheimer's Disease

- Reduce melatonin production (which is the most important detox agent for your brain and is also an anti-inflammatory).
- Promote breast cancer
- Miscarriage – 2x more likely
- Worsen inflammation by creating more potent mycotoxins; and reducing inflammation is vital

Mobile (cell) phones – Handsets give off microwaves which cause cells to mutate in a way which cannot be easily stopped. Researchers (Franz Aldkofer who led the 4 year £2.2 million study) found that cell mutation appeared to be more severe in older people. The findings of the EU-funded study showed that phone signals released highly reactive groups of free radicals which caused DNA to mutate. Furthermore, the new UMTS bandwidth is ten times more damaging to genes than GSM radiation. Reference: **http://www.next-up.org/pdf/PressReleaseConcernPrFranzAdelkofer VerumFoundation06102007.pdfU**

Cordless house phones – Unfortunately, these are just as damaging as cell phones. In fact, the newer phones using the 2.4 GHz frequencies are always on and therefore emitting even when no-one is talking on them.

WiFi (wireless internet signals) – these are, unfortunately, becoming more and more prevalent and radiate further than mobile phones. Their range is in fact more like cordless phones. If you live in a densely populated area like an apartment complex, then you are probably being subjected to several of these signals all the time.

Electric blankets & heating pads

This is a bigger threat than other household appliances. Electric blankets are capable of creating a magnetic field anywhere from *5 to 20 times higher* than the EPA's proposed safe level of exposure. Meanwhile, many scientists warn that these standards for electromagnetic exposures are too lax to protect human health. Electric blankets create a magnetic field that penetrates about 6-7 inches into your body – for hours at a time. This qualifies as chronic exposure.

Solutions include:

- o Distance is your best ally. The first and best course of action is to keep your distance from any electronic device while it is operating. Even a few feet makes a huge difference and after 10 feet, there is usually very little harmful effect.

- o The most important place to protect is your bed, because that's usually where you spend the most time and require the least disturbance. Therefore, remove all electrical wires that run under, behind, or even near your bed. That means move bedside lights further away and get a battery-powered bedside clock. If possible, move your bed so that the wall behind it (or near it) does not contain any internal wires.

- o In response to EMF concerns, U.S. electric blanket manufacturers now sell blankets that claim to generate no harmful electromagnetic radiation. Although these "zero magnetic field" blankets reduce or eliminate magnetic fields, they may still generate electric fields.

- EMFreedom.com can supply protective bed canopies that screen out 99.999% of these frequencies.

- **ZeroPoint pendant** - The ZeroPoint System works by creating a 3 to 5 foot "balancing" field around the body to offset the chaotic effects of EMF impact on our personal biofields wherever we are. ZeroPoint immediately neutralizes the effects of EMF and ELF waves in our bodies (and our foods). The main advantages with this is that it's easier to keep one of these pendants near your body than to install EMF screening, and of course the protection stays with you rather than just around your bed.
ZeroPoint Pendant
http://zpgv.zeropointglobal.com/products/packaging.shtml

Miscellaneous remedies

Earth contact

Incredibly simple as it may seem, contact with the Earth is very important for overall health and healing. This contact grounds the body by draining away stressful static electricity. Think about it: for the last few million years of our species' time on this planet, we've been outside, in the sunshine, and toiling on the bare Earth. Doesn't it make sense that our bodies are now so adapted that they require this element? The nice part is that it's absolutely free! So spend at least 5 minutes a day standing or lying with your bare skin directly on the Earth (not cement or roads). Technically, this drains out stressful static electricity. An even better grounding comes from getting in the salty ocean water, or at least some natural lake/pond/stream.

Flowers & plants

A new study published in Hort Technology has concluded that plants and flowers in hospital rooms really do have healing benefits, especially for patients who are recovering from surgery.

Ninety patients recovering form appendectomy were studied. They were assigned randomly to various hospital rooms, some with plants and some without. As they were recovering, the patients with plants in their rooms were in the company of eight different varieties of plants and flowers. Recovery time, heart rate level, temperature, blood pressure, perceived level of pain, fatigue and anxiety levels were measured.

According to the results, patients exposed to flowers and plants had quicker recovery from abdominal surgery, lower use of pain medication use, lower heart rates and decreased

www.wolfewellness.co

anxiety levels. The patients in rooms with plants were much more satisfied.

So you can now be especially grateful for those bouquets and plants.

Contact with a pet

It's a well-known fact that pet owners are happier, healthier, and live longer. So if you have room in your life for a pet, now's a good time. Of course, wait until you can get around comfortably first.

Get out of the hospital

Let's face it, hospitals are necessary, but most of them do not make for a good rehab environment. They are under constant threat of spreading contagious diseases, the psychic vibe in these places is usually quite heavy/negative/busy, and the EMF pollution is getting stronger all the time from the tech equipment they keep going 24 hours/day.

There's a common and very serious problem call Hospital Acquired Conditions (HAC) that runs as high as 30% in many US hospitals. This is where the patient picks up a new problem/disease from the hospital itself.

So be in the hospital for as long as you require critical treatments and special attention, then the sooner you can leave, the better. If possible for your particular operation, look for a local outpatient service instead of a full-blown hospital.

www.wolfewellness.co

Human contact

Touch therapy is a practice and art on its own. Laying-on-hands is an ancient healing art, but anyone can do it to some degree. Loved ones are obviously well suited to lend a hand. All massage is based on this premise of the healing power of touch. This is another good reason to go in for regular massage treatments. See the section on Massage for some suggestions.

Music & sound therapy

Although musical tastes vary widely, in clinical tests some music and sounds have been shown to offer much stronger healing benefits. It has been known for a long while that sounds and vibrations can have a huge impact on healing. There are many schools of therapy based on this knowledge and many people have received great benefit from it.

Organs and other body parts can be healed faster and emotions held in the organs can be released with greater ease and speed. The awakening and healing of your energy centers can also be sped up. Clearly, healing sounds can be very useful at this time when you desire better health.

Nature sounds such as birds, rainstorms, frogs or ocean waves, and various types of music, such as classical, are often used as a stress-relief tool. These sounds have a calming effect and can help patients to relax while undergoing medical procedures. Natural sounds and music have also been found to ease pain and reduce stress and anxiety while acting as mood enhancers.

What works well for many people is traditional instrumental/flute music. Also, a little-known fact is that music that follows 60 beats per minute is not only relaxing,

www.wolfewellness.co

but puts your brain in an alpha-wave state. There are many lovely baroque pieces that fit this bill.

Another simple rule of thumb to decide which music or sounds are best for you is to remember to use the ones that you are naturally drawn to.

Here's a very nice piece to add to your library. It uses binaural frequencies, which gently take you into a deeply meditative state and can have a direct healing and relaxing affect:
Sound healing with binaural frequencies

http://products.mercola.com/insight-focus/?aid=CD426

Just type **"music"** in the WellBasket search box

Sauna therapy

Heating of the tissues enhances metabolic processes. Greater cellular energy production facilitates healing. Viruses, tumors and toxin-laden cells are weaker than normal cells so they tolerate heat poorly. Therefore, raising the body temperature causes infections to heal more quickly. Saunas also enhance circulation and oxygenate the tissues. They open the nasal passages and assist the sinuses to drain. Although it's a major eliminative organ, most people's skin is very inactive - many do not sweat. Repeated use of the sauna slowly restores skin elimination. Toxic chemicals and metals can be removed faster than with any other method. It is a daily habit that pays many dividends.

Steam baths, sweat lodges, vigorous exercise and hot tubs are more extreme and less effective than far-infrared saunas. Far-infrared (as well as near-infrared) heats the body, while the air remains cool. Sweating begins quickly and the experience is rather pleasant. Preheating is unnecessary which saves electricity. According to research, far-infrared is more cleansing than traditional saunas. The deep penetration of the infrared energy allows the cells to eliminate better. If your budget can handle this expense, it is well worth it. Here's the right style sauna to achieve the above benefits.

Sauna

http://www.phmiracleliving.com/p-189-ph-miracle-dry-heat-sauna-model-1000.aspx?affiliateid=10152

Note that it's important to shower off the sweat ASAP coming out of the sauna so your body does not re-absorb the toxins it just excreted. Also, by using cool water, it locks in the warm energies and prevents you getting a chill afterwards. At some point when you're stronger, you can challenge and strengthen your immune system with cold baths as described by the Wim Hof Method.

Sleep

You heal while you sleep, so it makes sense to maximize its potential. Here is a list of useful tips:

- **Adrenals** – Have them checked by a good natural medicine clinician. Medical scientists have found that insomnia may be caused by adrenal stress (Journal of Clinical Endocrinology & Metabolism, August 2001; 86:3787-3794).
- **Alarm clocks** – If these devices must be used, keep them as far away from the bed as possible, preferably at least 3 feet because of electrical disturbance to you (see section on electromagnetic issues in this eBook). Better is a battery operated clock that only lights up when you press it So that its glow won't disturb you, as this will seriously impair your body's ability to produce melatonin. Loud alarm clocks are very stressful on the body by causing it to be awoken suddenly. If you are regularly getting enough sleep, they should be unnecessary. One solution is to use a sun alarm clock. **The Sun Alarm™ SA-2002** provides an ideal way to wake up each morning if you can't wake up with the REAL sun. Combining the features of a traditional alarm clock (digital display, AM/FM radio, beeper, snooze

button, etc) with a special built-in light that gradually increases in intensity, this amazing clock simulates a natural sunrise. It also includes a sunset feature where the light fades to darkness over time - ideal for anyone who has trouble falling asleep. In any case, it's best to ignore/hide this device as much as possible because it will only add to your worry when constantly staring at it... 2 a.m. ...3 a.m. ... 4:30 a.m.

- **Alcohol** – Although alcohol will make you drowsy, the effect is short lived and people will often wake up several hours later, unable to fall back asleep. Alcohol will also keep you from falling into the deeper stages of sleep, where the body does most of its healing.

- **Amount** – Get the right amount of sleep. The standard amount is between -9 hours. When you're recovering, it can be a little more, but also be careful not over-do sleep as that can make you lethargic and more prone to depression.

- **Bedroom** – Reserve your bed only for sleeping. If you are used to watching TV or doing work in bed, you may find it harder to relax there and to think of the bed as a place to sleep.

- **Caffeine** – Avoid. A recent study showed that in some people, caffeine is not metabolized efficiently and therefore they can feel the effects long after consuming it. So an afternoon cup of coffee (or even tea) will keep some people from falling asleep. Also, some medications, particularly diet pills contain caffeine.

- **Chi Gung (Qigong)** – In addition to its powerful healing techniques, Chi Gung will teach you how to deeply relax in a very short time. Here are a few unique and short examples from youtube. You will find many more with the simple search words: *chi gong for sleep.*
  - https://www.youtube.com/watch?v=xdb51q lCUyg&ab_channel=QiWithEli
  - https://www.youtube.com/watch?v=msjuEb tkA8o&ab_channel=TylerTrahan
  - https://www.youtube.com/watch?v=Sg6Z9b IAXq0&ab_channel=KristenPolzien
  - https://www.youtube.com/watch?v=QOpSR vy-BZY&ab_channel=QigongAwarenessLLC
  - https://www.youtube.com/watch?v=yyLWf-oNJT8&t=690s&ab_channel=ExerciseToHea l

- **Darkness** – Sleep in complete darkness or as close as possible. If there is even the tiniest bit of light in the room it can disrupt your circadian rhythm and your pineal gland's production of melatonin. There also should be as little light in the bathroom as possible if you get up in the middle of the night. Please whatever you do, keep the light off when you go to the bathroom at night. As soon as you turn on that light you will - for that night - immediately cease all production of the important sleep aid melatonin. Another solution is to have red lights in your bedroom/bathroom or a red flashlight during the night as that will not disrupt your melatonin flow.
- **Drugs** – Although over-the-counter (OTC) sleep drugs can get you to sleep, they can have unhealthy side-affects, especially with extended use.
- **EFT** – The Emotional Freedom Technique is very effective at inducing sleep. Go to that section in this eBook for further details.
- **EMFs** – Check your bedroom for electro-magnetic fields (EMFs). These can disrupt the pineal gland and the production of melatonin and seratonin, and may have other negative effects as well. To purchase a gauss meter to measure EMFs call Cutcat at 800-497-9516. They have a model for around $40. One doctor even recommends that people pull their circuit breaker before bed to kill all power in the house (Dr. Herbert Ross, author of "Sleep Disorders"). At a minimum, move your bed so that your head is at least 3-6 feet from all electrical outlets. There are also various bio-energetic protection devices, which I shall supply here in the next edition of this book.
- **Exercise** – At least a little exercise for at least 30 minutes everyday can help you rest better. However, don't exercise too close to bedtime or it may keep you awake. Studies show exercising in the morning or late afternoon (4pm – 7pm) is better.
- **Electrical devices and wires** – If any devices must be used, keep them as far away from the bed as possible, preferably at least 3 feet because of electrical disturbance to you (see section on electromagnetic issues in this eBook). So if you have electrical wires running under/near your bed – chances are they're disturbing your sleep.

- **Food** – Because people can react differently to eating, experiment with the following suggestions to find what works best for you.

- Eat a small piece of fruit. This can help the tryptophan cross the blood-brain barrier.
- Eat a (small) handful of walnuts before bed - they're a good source of tryptophan, a sleep-enhancing amino acid.
- Avoid foods that you may be sensitive to. This is particularly true for dairy and wheat products, as they may have effect on sleep, such as causing apnea, excess congestion, gastrointestinal upset, and gas, among others.
- Avoid grains and sugars. This will raise blood sugar and inhibit sleep. Later, when blood sugar drops too low (hypoglycemia), you might wake up and not be able to fall back asleep
- Full meals are generally poorly digested when you lie down, so finish any full meals within 4 hours of bedtime.

- **Fluids** – If you drink any fluids within 2 hours of going to bed, it will increase the need to go to the bathroom during the night.
- **Footsoak** – This was quite common practice in 50 some years ago. They often did this after a hard day because it can be a very soothing on your nervous system:

1. Get a plastic tub that can fit both your feet comfortably in a sitting position (I recommend a large, oval cleaning bucket as they're easier to handle)
2. Add a few tablespoons (each) of good quality salts:
   i. Sea salt – Himalayan and/or Dead Sea salts are excellent choices due to their added mineral content
   ii. Epsom salt – a traditional relaxing mineral
3. A few tablespoons of baking soda
4. A tablespoon of volcanic clay –bentonite or similar
5. 3-7 drops of lavender oil – increase relaxation
6. Fill the tub with warm water
7. Soak the feet for about 10 minutes. This is a good time to do a meditation with soothing music
8. Using a plastic pitcher near your chair, rinse feet with a little warm fresh water
9. Towel dry feet
10. Pour the water down the toilet, not the sink, because the water will have collected negative

energies that you would not want to affect eating utensils

- o Note also that an Ionic foot bath device is better still.
- **Fresh air** – Don't overlook the simple act of opening the window a bit. Your body rest better by maintaining oxygen levels during the night.

- **Gratitude** – Think of or write down about 3 things you're grateful for (and that you achieved) from that day or at this time… and allow yourself to *feel* grateful. This is proven by positive psychology studies to be very beneficial.

- **Herbs** – The following herbs help you to relax and, of course, sleep:
  - o California poppy
  - o Chamomile
  - o Kava Kava
  - o Lemon balm
  - o Lavender
  - o Oat milky seed
  - o Passion flower
  - o Skullcap
  - o Valerian root
  - o Wulinshen – helps you achieve deep delta sleep
- **Homeopathy** – Just as this can help with pain or other symptoms, homeopathic sleep formulae can work wonders for many people. With no side-effects, it is certainly worth using:
- **Hot bath, shower or sauna** 90 to 120 minutes before bed. It increases your core body temperature, and when it abruptly drops when you get out of the bath, it signals your body that you are ready for sleep.
- **Journaling** – If you often lay in bed with your mind racing, it might be helpful keep a journal and write down your thoughts before bed. If you wake in the middle of the night with your mind going, just transfer your to-do list or even current worries to the written page and then return to sleep -unworried. If you write about any stresses, it has now been proven to greatly reduce this stress and even alleviate certain conditions like asthma, arthritis, and others.
- **Listen to white noise or relaxation CDs** - Some people find the sound of white noise or nature sounds, such as the ocean or forest, to be soothing for sleep – even a low

humming fan or heater could help. However, to avoid too much of a good thing, put this sound on a timer so that it automatically turns off after 20-60 minutes.

- **Lose weight –** Being overweight can increase the risk of sleep apnea, which will prevent a restful nights sleep. If you follow a few of the dietary recommendations in this book, you will probably lose some weight.

- **Massage / spine –**
  - ○ Some people have chronic tension different body parts. So getting these parts relaxed with massage can really help (head, neck, shoulders, legs, etc).
  - ○ Here's where Cranial Sacral massage can relax the entire nervous system for deep sleep
  - ○ Also, if your top vertebrae (C1 at the base of skull) is out of place, then the whole body will be in an agitated state. A good chiropractor can help with this.

- **Melatonin –** This is a powerful hormone that is secreted by the pineal gland, a pea-size structure at the center of the brain. Its secretion is stimulated by the dark and inhibited by light. Melatonin helps our bodies regulate our sleep-wake cycles. Interestingly, the amount of melatonin produced by our body seems to lessen as we get older. Scientists believe this may be why young people have less problem sleeping than older people. Ideally it is best to increase levels naturally with exposure to bright sunlight in the daytime (along with full spectrum fluorescent bulbs in the winter) and absolute complete darkness at night. You should get blackout drapes so no light is coming in from the outside. You can also use one of melatonin's precursors, L-tryptophan which is the safe and effective, but must be obtained by prescription only. However, don't be afraid or intimidated by its prescription status. It is just a simple amino acid. Melatonin usage:

  - ○ Suggested amounts vary from 0.5 – 5 milli-grams. You'll need to experiment to find out your own ideal dosage.

  - ○ Take about 30 minutes before bed. But remember, not with a big glass of water or you'll be back in the bathroom long before morning.

- **Menopausal or perimenopausal –** Get checked out by a good natural medicine physician. The hormonal changes at this time may cause problems if not properly addressed.

- **Pets** – Dogs, cats, and other pets in your bed can provide emotional support, but weigh this against the distraction of them snoring, shifting, or disturbing your own sleep states.
- **Move your bed away from outside walls,** which will help cut down on noise.
- **Music** – Play some gentle, soothing music before going to bed or put your player on a timer for about 10-30 minutes when you lie down. What works well for many people is traditional instrumental/flute music. Also, music that follows 60 beats per minute is not only relaxing, but puts your brain in an alpha-wave state.
- **Pillows** – Choose the right one and don't skimp here because you spend a third of your life in bed (and even more during recovery).
  - Neck pillows, which resemble a rectangle with a depression in the middle, can enhance the quality of your sleep and reduce neck pain. A simple rule is that it's better to have a lower pillow than one that's too high.
  - To check your unique size requirement, lie on your side and have someone look at your spine: your head & neck should be exactly level with the rest of your back.

- **Read** something spiritual or religious. This will help to relax. Don't read anything stimulating, such as a mystery or suspense novel, as this may have the opposite effect. In addition, if you are really enjoying a suspenseful book, you might wind up unintentionally reading for hours, instead of going to sleep.
- **Socks** – Experiment with wearing socks to bed.
  - Because they have the poorest circulation, the feet often feel cold before the rest of the body. A study has shown that this reduces night wakings. Warm feet -- a sign of healthy blood flow -- may help induce restful sleep. So warming up cold feet, such as with an old-fashioned hot water bottle, could help those who have trouble falling asleep. Thermoregulation -- the body's heat distribution system -- is strongly linked to sleep cycles. Even lying down increases sleepiness by redistributing heat in the body from the core to the periphery.
  - On the other hand, after some hours of sleep, some people need to cool down, so having the feet too

warm can interrupt sleep. As with many things, people have different needs at different times. So experiment with this practice.

- **Sprinkle sheets and pillowcases with lavender** – This scent is proven to promote relaxation. You can either put some drops on your pillow or place a little sack of dried lavender near your head. It's also a good idea to wash bed linen about every 1-2 weeks.
- **Sunlight** – Yes, getting a full dose of blazing sunlight during the day will help your body regulate its biorhythms at night.
- **Temperature** – Many people keep their bedrooms too hot for good sleep. The ideal temperature should be around 65 degrees F. If this is a big, uncomfortable change, then slowly reduce the temperature a little bit each night to re-adjust your body.

- ## Timing –

  - Everyone needs at least 7 hours every night and most should not sleep over 9 hours. During recovery, this might be a little longer, but come back into this range soon after the Inflammatory stage is over.

  - Don't change your bedtime. You should go to bed, and wake up, at the same times each day, even on the weekends. This will help your body to get into a sleep rhythm and make it easier to fall asleep and get up in the morning.

  - Establish a bedtime routine. This could include meditation, deep breathing, a massage from your partner, and the suggestions in this section. The key is to find what makes you feel relaxed, then repeat it each night.

  - Our systems, particularly the adrenals, do a majority of their recharging or recovering during the hours of 11 p.m. and 1 a.m. In addition, your gallbladder dumps toxins during this same period. If you are awake, the toxins back up into the liver which then secondarily back up into your entire system and cause further disruption of your health. Prior to the widespread use of electricity, people would go to bed shortly after sundown, as most animals do, and which nature intended for humans as well. Some people have very different timing preferences, but the normal circadian rhythm suggests that around 10pm is ideal.

- o Afternoon naps are generally good for most people, however, they can also be a source of insomnia. During recovery stages you will probably be resting/sleeping much more.

- **TV** – Avoid watching TV before bed (within at least 1 hour). Even better, get the TV out of the bedroom completely. The white and blue light is too stimulating to the pineal gland and causes it to not produce natural melatonin on time, and it will then take longer to fall asleep.
- **Vitamin B** – B12 & B6 are popular, but it's usually better to take the entire complex as they synergistically improve each other. You can take these during the day or before bed...see which way feels better.
- **Wear an eye mask to block out light** – As said above, it is very important to sleep in as close to complete darkness as possible. However, it's not always easy to block out every stream of light using curtains, blinds or drapes, particularly if you live in an urban area (or if your spouse has a different schedule than you do). In these cases, a sleep mask can help to block out the remaining light.
- **Work** – Put your work away at least one hour (but preferably two or more) before bed. This will give your mind a chance to unwind so you can go to sleep feeling calm.
- **Military trick** to help you fall asleep in a few minutes. After just six weeks of practice, 96% of pilots could fall asleep within 120 seconds. Credit to Aaron Smith, Quora (https://qr.ae/pGqNI1).
  - o If it works for combat pilots, it will work for you, regardless of how stressed you are about that meeting tomorrow.

1. Breathe slowly and deeply, relaxing the muscles in your face. Release any tension in your forehead, jaw, and around your eyes. **Hint:** a little facial massage goes a long way.
2. Relax your body. Start with your shoulders, dropping them as low as possible. Then loosen your upper and lower arm on one side and then the other.

 www.wolfewellness.co

3. While breathing in deeply and exhaling slowly, relax your upper body and then release any tension in your legs, from your thighs to your lower legs.
4. After your entire body has relaxed for 10 seconds, clear your mind. This can be done by doing one of the following:
   - Imagine yourself lying in a canoe on a serene lake with blue sky above you.
   - Picture yourself all cozy and warm in a black velvet hammock in a pitch-black room.
   - Rewind/review your entire day as best you can back to the moment you awoke that day (Greg's improved version).
5. Once you are physically relaxed and your mind is empty for at least 10 seconds, you'll probably fall asleep.
6. Within minutes, you'll be out like a light. Remember 96% of combat pilots achieved success after six weeks of practice. These weeks of practice are a worthwhile investment, because once you have it down, you can nap and sleep anywhere, which will dramatically improve your quality of life.
7. These are great exercises not only for sleep, but they work extremely well for chronic pain.

Sunlight

- This is another essential remedy. The good news is that if you live in a sunny place, it's a free and pleasant treatment.
- The beneficial ultraviolet rays of the sun get filtered out before the others that can burn your skin. The simplest and best way to choose when to sun-bathe is on a clear day when your own shadow is no longer than your own height. Otherwise, the best rays are not available at that time.
- It is important to stress that you should never get burned and should only implement sun exposure very gradually. You will know you've had enough sunlight when your skin turns the lightest shade of pink. It can take 3-6 times longer for darker pigmented skin to reach the equilibrium concentration of skin pre vitamin D. However, skin pigmentation does not affect the amount of vitamin D that can be obtained through sunshine exposure. Beyond that you're only increasing your risk of getting burned, which can cause skin damage. An equilibrium occurs in white

www.wolfewellness.co

skin (with at least 40% surface area) within 20 min of ultraviolet exposure, at which point further increases in vitamin D is not possible, because the ultraviolet light will start to degrade the vitamin D. At least once/week is needed and up to once/day is good. Needless to say, most people are very deficient in this.

- Sunlight forms on the surface of your skin and then takes several hours for the body to fully absorb the vitamin D3 into the blood stream. Realizing how our bodies have evolved over the last 2 million years, it's important not to shower off the large areas of your body with soap. This means it's ok to soap those areas that form bacteria (under arms and groin area) but just don't use soap (soon after sun bathing) on your back, chest and legs so that you can allow most of the D3 in natural skin oil to be absorbed.
- Before considering supplementation with vitamin D, it would be wise to have your vitamin D level tested. This is best done from a nutritionally oriented physician. It is very important that they order the correct test. The advantage of having your medical doctor perform the test is that it will usually be covered by your medical insurance.
- The best vitamin D test is 25(OH)D (also called 25-hydroxyvitamin D). It is this marker that is most strongly associated with overall health. Please note the difference between normal and optimal. You don't want to be average here; you want to be optimally healthy.
- Here is test kit from the Vitamin D Council that you can order:
  http://www.vitamindcouncil.org/health/deficiency/am-i-vitamin-d-deficient.shtml
- It's imperative that you find out if your lab has performed the appropriate recalibrations against Liaison's (DiaSorin's) assays. Otherwise your vitamin D levels may be vastly overstated, in some cases by as much as 40 percent, meaning you may get the green light that your levels are fine, when in fact you are deficient, or perhaps even dangerously low.
- If you have sarcoidosis, tuberculosis, or lymphoma, it would be best for you to avoid oral vitamin D supplementation based on this test. It is recommended that you perform the 1,25(OH)D test before you supplement with any sun exposure or oral vitamin D as it is a better indicator in people with this health challenge.

Mind-body connection

You've probably heard of some miraculous recoveries from people using prayer, positive thinking, or other mental/spiritual methods. Your mind (and heart) has incredible power to make your body strong and whole. Here are a few structured ways for you to begin to reap the rewards of this treasure.

Autosuggestion technique

Step1
Look for a comfortable, quiet location where you won't experience any interruptions or distractions.

Step2
Try to clear your mind of all thoughts. This will be difficult at first. It will get easier with practice. When thoughts do enter your mind, take a moment to simply observe, witness, and acknowledge them. Let them pass.

Step3
Focus on the tense points in your body. You'll need to know exactly where you're carrying tension and stress in order to make yourself fully relaxed.

Step4
Take slow deep breaths and focus on releasing the tension in your identified places. As you inhale, imagine a bright light filling that area with energy, or life force. As you exhale, imagine the tension as dark, inky smoke coming from the wound and out of your mouth and nose.

Step5
Count backwards from 10 when you feel truly relaxed. It may help for you to imagine each number in your head as you're counting.

 www.wolfewellness.co

Step6
Create a positive statement about your upcoming or recent surgery. Your statement can be just about anything, as long as it has to do with a positive aspect of your speedy recovery.

Step7
Repeat your statement several times until you feel your mind responding to this suggestion.

Step8
When you're ready to return to an alert and energetic state, just count from 0 to 10. Give yourself a moment to adjust to normal consciousness.

If you are lucky enough to be reading this book before your surgery, then have your doctor say a few positive healing words about you and your recovery *during your surgery, while you are unconscious*.

Visualization

Visualizing is when you use your mind to imagine how things (or your body) could be. There is now irrefutable evidence as to the power that your mind has over your body. In fact, you are visualizing something about yourself and/or a future outcome nearly all the time. Learning to harness this powerful resource to become a source of healing is an invaluable skill – many people have a negative self-image and that is damaging in many ways.

Learning to visualize positively could be a silver lining of your recovery experience. Because learning this activity could take up an entire book on its own, I recommend you find an audio that is appropriate for your condition, and/or allow an expert to lead you on this aspect of recovery.

 www.wolfewellness.co

EFT (Emotional Freedom Technique)

EFT stands for "*Emotional Freedom Techniques*" and is an easy and amazingly fast "tapping" technique. You just lightly but firmly tap on certain acupuncture/acupressure points on the face, head and upper body and astonishing events begin to take place. The process quickly and easily activates the body's own "energy meridian system" and has great potential for releasing virtually anything that's "wrong" with you.

EFT has been shown to provide relief from:

- chronic pain
- emotional problems
- disorders
- addictions
- phobias
- post traumatic stress disorder
- physical issues

And all this with no side effects!

While EFT and the use of "energy systems" in general is somewhat new to the Western world, it is set to revolutionize the field of health and wellness by using healing concepts that have been in practice in Eastern medicine for over 5,000 years.

Chi Gung (Qigong)

This method works on both the mind-body connection and gentle physical exercise. It is a very direct and powerful healing method that is the highest healing practice developed over many centuries in China.

www.wolfewellness.co

Please refer to this same sub-heading in the Physical Exercise section for complete details or more information about Qigong.

Sedona Method: A simple exercise

We are all either our own worst enemy or our own best friend. We are constantly sabotaging our health, happiness, and success unintentionally due to our unresolved thinking, beliefs, and attitudes. Yet even when we know a thought, belief or attitude is not serving us, most of us find it very difficult to change it or let it go. The reason for this problem is very simple: our emotions color, create, and lock these limitations in place, making the limitations supposedly "real." It is our emotions that either put us into action or prevent us from acting. The Sedona Method will show you how to master your emotions, thereby mastering how you think and act. That is the short explanation of why this one technique can influence your recovery process – in addition to many other areas.

Let me explain further by asking you to participate in a simple exercise. Pick up a pen, a pencil, or some small object that you would be willing to drop without giving it a second thought. Now, hold it in front of you and really grip it tightly. Pretend this is one of your limiting feelings and that your hand represents your gut or your consciousness. If you held the object long enough, this would start to feel uncomfortable yet familiar.

Now, open your hand and roll the object around in it. Notice that you are the one holding on to it; it is not attached to your hand. The same is true with your feelings, too. Your feelings are as attached to you as this object is attached to your hand.

  www.wolfewellness.co

We hold on to our feelings and forget that we are holding on to them. It's even in our language. When we feel angry or sad, we don't usually say, "I feel angry," or, "I feel sad." We say, "I am angry," or, "I am sad." Without realizing it, we are misidentifying that we are the feeling. Often, we believe a feeling is holding on to us. This is not true... we are always in control and just don't know it.

Now, let the object go.

What happened? You let go of the object, and it dropped to the floor. Was that hard? Of course not. That's what we mean when we say "let go."

You can do the same thing with any emotion: choose to let it go.

　　　www.wolfewellness.co

Dealing with the pain

Although there are numerous techniques and therapies to reduce pain, this section lists those focused on methods that are quick for you to learn and also heal you, not just reduce the discomfort. It's also important to realize that although you want to ease the pain immediately, it is a signal to you that something is not yet right in your body. So improving your overall health will insure that you heal the problem, and then the pain will vanish by itself. This means follow the guidelines in each main section of this book to heal faster and completely.

For engaging your mind-over-body controls, see the appropriate sections for details on the following techniques:

- Acupressure & Acupuncture
- Chi Gung (Qigong)
- EFT
- Sedona Method – also see excerpt below
- Visualization

Herbs for pain

Not surprisingly, the list of herbs to help reduce pain and inflammation are similar to those that help you sleep.

- **Boswellia** - An ingredient used for thousands of years, current research shows that Boswellia serrata supports the body's own anti-inflammatory response. Recent investigations also suggest that inhibition of inflammatory compounds in the body may also provide support of healthy cell development.

www.wolfewellness.co

- **California poppy -** This pain reliever is also a good sedative for headaches and insomnia with no toxic side effects. It is commonly used as an infusion in tinctures and dried powder of herbs in helping ease the pain. While closely related to opium poppy, it has the opposite effect. Instead of disrupting your psychological orientation, it stabilizes it.

- **Cayenne-capsicum (cream) –**this form of cayenne helps to alleviate pain by depleting the body's supply of substance P, a chemical component of nerve cells that transmits pain signals to the brain.

- **Chamomile -** One of the safest medicinal herbs, chamomile is a soothing, gentle relaxant that has been shown to work for a variety of complaints from stress to menstrual cramps. Although best known as a muscle relaxant and antispasmodic, chamomile also has antiseptic and anti-inflammatory capabilities. Chamomile has been shown to promote general relaxation and relieve stress. Animal studies show that chamomile contains substances that act on the same parts of the brain and nervous system as anti-anxiety drugs. Chamomile also helps to control insomnia.

- **Ginger –** Fresh ginger has been proven as a pain and natural anti-inflammatory remedy.

- **Kava Kava -** A member of the lamiaceae family, the Skullcap plant has a long history of use in the western Naturopathic Tradition. It was used to support exhausted nerves resulting from mental and physical exhaustion, maintain normal balance in times of muscular tension, and support normal sleep patterns. Many Eclectic Medical texts mention its use to support the nerves during withdrawl from drugs. It is trophorestorative to the nervous system meaning it restores nutrition uptake to the nerves.

   www.wolfewellness.co

Like most mints it is cooling yet has bitter principles and other complex chemicals making it a balanced choice as a gentle nervine.

- **Lavender** - is most often found in soaps, shampoos, and aromatics due to its wonderful scent; in fact, the name lavender comes from the Latin root lavare, which means "to wash." Lavender most likely earned this name because it was frequently used in baths to help purify the body and spirit. However, this herb is also considered a natural remedy for a range of ailments from insomnia and anxiety to depression and mood disturbances. Recent studies prove hundreds of years of anecdotal evidence showing that lavender produces calming, soothing, and sedative effects. There is now scientific evidence to suggest that lavender slows the activity of the nervous system, improves sleep quality, promotes relaxation, and lifts mood in people suffering from pain disorders. Lavender has even been approved by Germany's Commission E (similar to our FDA) as a treatment for insomnia, restlessness, and nervous stomach irritations

- **Lemon balm** - doesn't come from lemons; rather, it is a lemon scented member of the mint family. As far back as the ancient Greeks this plant was recognized for both its soothing smell and its medicinal properties. The Greek physician Dioscorides would apply lemon balm to scorpion or animal bites for its antibacterial properties, and then give the patient wine infused with lemon balm to calm their nerves. This calming affect has often been noted throughout the years. The esteemed British herbalist Nicholas Culpeper said in the mid-1600s "[lemon balm] causeth the mind and heart to be Merry...and driveth away all troublesome cares." It has a slightly sedative effect, and can be helpful in lowering fever,

www.wolfewellness.co

relaxing spasms and improving digestion. In 2003 researchers in the United Kingdom found that it can also help strengthen long-term memory.

- **Oat milky seed** - also contains B-complex vitamins. Most of the published research on Avena sativa has been conducted on the rolled or prepared oats, beta-glucans and fiber contained in the oat. The relaxing properties of minerals on tissues is well noted and at least worth considering when attempting to explain a plant's ability to calm restless nerves.

- **Passionflower** - has a depressant effect on the activity of the central nervous system. It is used for its sedative and soothing properties, to lower blood pressure, prevent tachycardia and for insomnia. Passion flower has recently been shown to have sedative activity in animals.

- **Skullcap** - is a nervine and contains numerous flavanoids and flavones including the flavanoid glycoside Scutellarin, essential oils, tannins, and iridoids. Scutellarin acts like quercitin in that it decreases mast cell activity.

- **Valerian root** - The plant was so valued in medieval times as a pain and relaxant remedy, that it was known by the name, "All Heal." Its ability to help relax the central nervous system, promote feelings of calm, decrease levels of anxiety and stress, and enhance sleep are known to millions the world over. Unlike some prescription aids, valerian is not known to cause grogginess and is non-addictive.

- **White willow bark** – its key ingredient is salicin, a glycoside that is converted into salicylic acid by the liver. Salicylic acid from white willow supports healthy levels of prostaglandins, compounds generated by the COX pathway and involved in the body's natural anti-inflammatory response. It is also the key ingredient in conventional aspirin, however, when taken in its whole-herb form it is much gentler on the stomach and liver.

Don't forget that enzymes – while they may not give fast-acting relief – also reduce pain in the long term. See the section on enzymes for more details.

For localized aches and pains, a combination of essential oils and DMSO can make an effective topical formula. When you do this, be sure that the essential oils are organic and approved for internal use.

Homeopathic remedies to reduce pain

The follow list is by no means complete, but it will help guide you to some good sources:

- Arnica Montana – painful limbs, joints, injuries, sprains

- Beladonna – neuralgia, throbbing headaches, sharp pains

- Gelsemium sempervirens – pain in hips, shoulders, back, muscles

- Gnaphalium polycephalum – sciatica, leg/joint pains, cramps

- Magnesia Phosphorica – muscle cramps, radiating pains, neuralgia

- Sanguinaria Canadensis – headache, pain in temples, eyes, back

- Salix alba – headache, muscle pain, back

Also, see the other Homeopathic section in this book.

www.wolfewellness.co

The emotional secret to overcoming physical pain – Sedona excerpt

Your mind and your body are intricately connected. This is why upon ending a relationship your heart can feel like it's breaking. It's also why your nerves can manifest into nausea, sweating or trembling hands.

Research shows that stress and other negative emotions can weaken your immune system, leaving you vulnerable to colds, flu and other infections. In fact, after a serious loss, such as a death in the family, the emotional jolt is severe enough to increase your risk of death.

"There is an increased risk of dying in the six months after bereavement and it's particularly marked amongst men," Martin Cowie, professor of cardiology at the Brompton Hospital, said in a BBC News article.

It's thought that the increased risk comes from the stress hormones surging during this time, which increase your risk of heart attacks and stroke.

Numerous other studies also show strong ties between emotions and physical illness or pain. For instance, a study by Naomi Eisenberger at the University of California, Los Angeles (UCLA) found that the pain of being socially rejected was processed by the brain in much the same way as physical pain, and in the same area, the anterior cingulate cortex.

Abraham Hicks, who lectures on the ideas behind the Law of Attraction, has been quoted as saying, "Physical pain is just an extension of emotion. It's all the same thing. There are two emotions. One feels good and one feels bad."

While negative emotions are capable of causing you physical pain, the opposite also holds true: positive emotions can help you ease and overcome physical pain.

www.wolfewellness.co

Positive Emotions Can Help You Overcome Physical Pain

Anthony Ong, assistant professor of human development at Cornell University, has conducted studies to determine how emotional states of mind influence physical and mental well-being. What he found was that people in a healthy state of mind could choose to focus on their positive emotions, and in so doing possibly heal faster and ease their pain.

Similarly, a review of studies by Robert Kerns, Ph.D. of the VA Connecticut Healthcare System found that psychological interventions helped patients with back pain to improve related depression and quality of life, and also to reduce their experience of pain.

This is why, if you are currently suffering from any type of physical pain, tending to your emotions is essential, and The Sedona Method is a highly recommended tool to help you do so.

"Although suffering associated with physical pain has an emotional component, when we feel like it is our pain and we compare the pain we're feeling now to our other pains, the sensations are magnified exponentially," says Hale Dwoskin, CEO and director of training of Sedona Training Associates. "In other words, when we resist what we're feeling we suffer accordingly."

This is because the more you resist, fear, or dread the pain, the more you are drawing pain into your experience. Even waking up in the morning and thinking "I'm tired of feeling pain all day" could be enough to manifest more pain into your life.

However, if you wake up and accept what is, without worrying or even thinking about pain, you will be preparing yourself to expect, and to have, a pain-free day.

"The Sedona Method can help you let go of all the emotions and memories tied to what you are experiencing physically," Dwoskin says. "There are two great ways to do this. First, you can experiment with welcoming the sensations that you are labeling pain and also welcome the emptiness or space on or in which those sensations are appearing. If you are not aware of emptiness or space you can simply welcome the parts of your body that are sensation-free."

"Another great way to release pain is to welcome the sensations and then look through the labels to what is here now," Dwoskin says. "As soon as you've labeled a sensation as pain, you are relating to what was, more than to what is. By rediscovering what is here now, pain often dissolves."

To get an idea of how this can be put into action, check out their main website (https://www.sedona.com/Home.asp).

Bringing it all together – recommended schedule

There is obviously a lot of information in this book that describes many things you can and should do to reclaim your health at this critical juncture. The following table will help by giving you an idea of what to do and when to do it. Note that if you got this book after having a surgery, then you should still read and consider some of the items in the preparatory stage, especially environmental items. You'll notice that some of these stages overlap. This means that your body might, for instance, be dealing with prolonged inflammation even as it is rebuilding surrounding tissues – so just use your discretion and intuition as to whether you are well enough to begin the suggestions from the later stage.

www.wolfewellness.co

Healing Stage	Nutrition	Physical & Environmental	Mind-Body
1. Pre-surgery (up to 8 weeks before surgery)	• Super healing drink – daily • Adjust diet towards whole, raw foods • Omega-3 supplements (discontinue this for the 7 days before surgery) • Vitamin C (4-10 grams/day except only ½ gram within 3 days before surgery) • Antioxidants – turmeric • Digestive enzymes • Proper hydration – see *Water* section • Begin SinEcch homeopathic remedy a day before surgery • Minimize/eliminate sugars and high-glycemic foods • Avoid harmful foods and influences as noted in *Avoid* sections • Cut back on Omega-6 oils	• Examine your home and bed to reduce EMF & geopathic disturbances • Get an appropriate cold/hot pack • Locate and sample some effective massage therapists • Begin an enjoyable exercise routine – especially develop those areas that will be affected by the operation • Prepare a close friend to help cope with situations that you think could happen • Sun bathing – or better, exercise in the sun & barefoot on the earth • Trampoline/rebounding exercise • Learn Chi-gung • Rest well for at least the 2 days before surgery	• Begin learning at least one method from this area: • EFT, Sedona Method, Chi-gung • Consider getting a loving pet • Get an appropriate visualization CD or script • Locate a source of laughter (people, movies, games) • Select healing music • Locate supportive friends and groups who have endured similar challenges

135

Healing Stage	Nutrition	Physical & Environmental	Mind-Body
2. Wound sealing (1-5 days after) & **Inflammatory** (1-21 days after)	• Proteolytic Enzymes • SinEcch homeopathic remedy • Super healing drink – daily • Dietary needs will vary according to your condition. At least take a few glasses of fresh-squeezed juices • Continue diet of whole, raw foods as per the section *Food* & general diet concepts • Omega-3 supplements • Reduce foods containing Omega-6 oils: proteins should be more from fish and a little grass-fed beef • Antioxidant fruits: berrys, grapes, plums • Vitamins: multi, C, E, D, K • Probiotics	• Use your cold pack to cool the inflamed area • If possible, do the Elephant Swing at least 2x/day • Chi-gung exercises: very important! • Gentle walking and stretching, as much as allowable • Try acupuncture to help reduce pain and discomfort • Follow enough of the sleep suggestions to achieve deep rest • Try some of the remedies from the *Miscellaneous* section to find what suits you best • Avoid heaving lifting as appropriate for your condition • Self-massage around the wound without disturbing it	• Use your visualization technique or CD • Use at least 1 of the methods you've chosen from: EFT and/or Sedona Release Method • Laugh often! • Share your successes with support network

www.wolfewellness.co

Healing Stage	Nutrition	Physical & Environmental	Mind-Body
2. Wound sealing (1-5 days after) & **Inflammatory** (1-21 days after)	• Minerals: Selenium, Zinc • Proper hydration – see *Water* section • Minimize sugars and high-glycemic foods • Select meats that are grass-fed organic • Select organic poultry that is pasture raised • Reduce dairy fat – especially when not raw & not from grass-fed animals • Avoid harmful foods and influences as noted in *Avoid* sections Contraindication: if you must take anti-inflammatory or blood-thinning medications, then do not take it with vit E, aloe vera, garlic, ginger, or fish oil. •	• When the wound has sealed and bandages are no longer required, then self-massage with the home-made formula as much as possible as discussed in section, *Self massage on outer scar tissue*	•

www.wolfewellness.co

Healing Stage	Nutrition	Physical & Environmental	Mind-Body
3. Tissue building (4-90 days after)	• Continue diet from previous stage and modify as follows: • Increase grass-fed beef if desired, continue with fish • Continue avoiding harmful foods such as omega 6 oils, refined carbs, chemically treated foods	• Begin alternating warmth with cold if inflammation is down • Continue Chi-gung • Exercise should become more vigorous – consider trampoline as appropriate • Consider other massages as appropriate and locally available • Lymph drainage and circulating massage • Self-massage closer to the wound without disturbing it – use your discretion with the pressure • When you can shower, use the hot/cold shower method	• Continue with the methods established in the prior stage that work for you

www.wolfewellness.co

Healing Stage	Nutrition	Physical & Environmental	Mind-Body
4. Matrix reforming (3 mos – 3 years)	• Continue diet from previous stage and modify as follows: • Phase in more poultry as desired – within dietary guidelines discussed • Reduce Vit C to 3000 mg/day • Reduce Vit E to 400 iu/day •	• Use more warmth to stimulate circulation and regrowth • Continue Chi-gung • Exercise should become more vigorous – consider trampoline as appropriate • Sleep patterns should come back to the normal range – as explained in the *Sleep* section	• Adjust your lifestyle so that you enjoy healthy choices more than quick fixes – the Sedona Method will help you with this

Personal Support

If you've come this far, then you are indeed determined to recover from that mishap/surgery/illness, and after digesting some of this book, you will bounce back better than ever! However, even though this book is a big download, the volume of new advances and knowledge is growing every day, so there is 10x more than this simple overview can contain.

It's obvious that conventional medical technologies are constantly improving, but they are mainly focused on crises intervention. *So after pulling someone out of an acute* (sometimes life-threatening) situation, they offer little to help you to regain or improve your health. In the same way, natural healing remedies are also making exponential advances from 1000s of specialists. Taking advantage of these latest natural, holistic-based healing technologies is an entirely different specialty…. that's where this program fits in.

Personal support is the way to get superior, faster, and long-term health gains. That means this could be the most important section for you.

Who needs personal support, and who is the right fit for this program?

- Fast and more complete wound healing
- Re-establishing your systemic stamina for a robust body, mind, and emotional state
- Weight issues – obesity increases risk of early death (heart attack, diabetes, etc, …)

www.wolfewellness.co

- Embarrassing skin issues that destroy self-esteem and restrict lifestyle
- Energy – reverse chronic or acute low energy levels so you can bounce out of bed and skip through your day like a teenager
- Mood & emotions – increase positive feelings that will bring joy to your life and all those around you
- Joints – reduce pain, inflammation, and stiffness
- Pain – relieve intense or chronic pain which decreases length/quality of life
- Strength – increase in specific areas and general stamina
- Vitality – recover the bounce of youth
- Chronic diseases
- Acute diseases
- Toxic sick feelings
- Lack of joy of living

www.wolfewellness.co

How personal support works

For me to understand your unique needs, here is my high-level consulting sequence.

1. You schedule an initial free call with me to get acquainted and see if this is the right fit for you
2. You fill out the health coaching client intake questionnaire to identify your initial needs, background, and profile
3. We conduct a custom analysis of your:
   - Current state of health
   - Health challenges
   - Relevant history
   - Personal factors
   - Environmental factors
   - Bio-marker analysis
4. We prioritize your needs
5. We create a custom plan for your elevating journey
6. We form a partnership to ensure you get to experience and benefit from the very best healing methodologies, technologies, and biological input that is currently available
7. I support you to monitor, assess, and adjust your dynamic healing experience for ever better results

Standard personal support

- Included in the primary personal support, I also offer:
  - Customized guidance to acquire the needed supplements, foods, and equipment
  - Energy healing sessions focused on your needs
  - Discussion and introduction to healing technologies that are relevant to you

www.wolfewellness.co

      o   Warm guidance from a genuine connection with your new healing support team!

Premium personal support

- For those who want to gain more from their healthspan and lifespan coaching, I can also engage with you further to create a custom-curated experience to include the following first-class longevity protocols:
  - o Personalized assistance obtaining required supplements, foods, and equipment
  - o Energy healing sessions - as logistically feasible
  - o Personally guided introductions to powerful rejuvenating technologies, treatments, and exclusive healing centers
  - o Top-tier analysis and cleansing treatments
  - o Warm support from genuine connections with like-minded community!

Results you can expect

- Enjoy more high-energy activities with your entire family and friends for many years to come
- Live long and energetic years to play with your great-grandkids
- Experience more and higher quality sex with your partner (think more energy and bonus connection tips)
- Higher quality of life – feeling great!
- Increased self-confidence in your body image and emotional state
- Increased productivity to crush your goals
- Better alignment with soul path
- Stabilize your ideal weight

www.wolfewellness.co

- Create a healthy and joyful lifestyle while having fun
- Enjoy spontaneous compliments about your new youthful radiance

What's needed from you to make this program work

- Motivation to change
- Some time to learn
- Adjustments to your lifestyle

Next steps and how to start personal coaching

Contact me via any of these methods to take advantage of an initial free consulting call.

- www.wolfewellness.co

- greg@wolfewellness.co

- https://calendly.com/gregww/30min

References

1. Water: https://www.mayoclinic.org/healthy-lifestyle/nutrition-and-healthy-eating/in-depth/water/art-20044256

2. Water: https://www.yogiapproved.com/health-wellness/how-to-drink-water-stay-hydrated-the-ayurvedic-way/

3. Ody, P, The Complete Medicinal Herbal, DK Publishing, New York, 1993

4. Christopher, JR, School of Natural Healing, Utah, 1999 (11th printing)

5. Herb Allure Nutritional Research, Jamestown, article on Garlic

6. Christopher, JR, School of Natural Healing, Utah, 1999 (11th printing)

7. Dr. Robert O. Young, The pH Miracle

8. Dr. Jon Baron, Lessons From The Miracle Doctors, and various articles

9. Dr. Joseph Mercola, various articles

10. Cohen M, Wolfe R, Mai T, et al. A randomized, double blind, placebo controlled trial of a topical cream containing glucosamine sulfate, chondroitin sulfate, and camphor for osteoarthritis of the knee. *J Rheumatol*. 2003 Mar;30(3):523-8.

11. Knuesel O, Weber M, Suter A. Arnica montana gel in osteoarthritis of the knee: an open, multicenter clinical trial. *Adv Ther*. 2002 Sep-Oct;19(5):209-18.

12. Sosa S, Altinier G, Politi M, et al. Extracts and constituents of Lavandula multifida with topical anti-inflammatory activity.*Phytomedicine*. 2005 Apr;12(4):271-7.

13. HBOT, https://www.hopkinsmedicine.org/health/treatment-tests-and-therapies/hyperbaric-oxygen-therapy#:~:text=HBOT%20helps%20wound%20healing%20by,and%20tissue%20starts%20to%20die

14. Laser and red light therapy, https://www.webmd.com/skin-problems-and-treatments/red-light-therapy

15. Daily JW, Yang M, Park S. Efficacy of Turmeric Extracts and Curcumin for Alleviating the Symptoms of Joint Arthritis: A Systematic Review and Meta-Analysis of Randomized Clinical Trials. J Med Food. 2016;19(8):717-729. doi:10.1089/jmf.2016.3705

16. Peterson CT, Vaughn AR, Sharma V, et al. Effects of Turmeric and Curcumin Dietary Supplementation on Human Gut Microbiota: A Double-Blind, Randomized, Placebo-Controlled Pilot Study. J Evid Based Integr Med. 2018;23:2515690X18790725. doi:10.1177/2515690X18790725

17. 10 Power Foods For Healing Wounds, https://www.organicfacts.net/home-remedies/foods-for-healing-wounds.html